Modern Neuromuscular Techniques

For Churchill Livingstone:

Commissioning editor: Inta Ozols
Project development editor: Valerie Bain
Project manager: Valerie Burgess
Project controller: Derek Robertson
Design direction: Judith Wright
Copy editor: Stephanie Pickering
Sales promotion executive: Maria O'Connor

Modern Neuromuscular Techniques

Leon Chaitow ND DO
Practitioner and Senior Lecturer,
University of Westminster, London, UK

Judith (Walker) DeLany LMT (Chapter 11: American neuromuscular techniques)
Director of NeuroMuscular Therapy Training Center,
St Petersburg, Florida, USA

Illustrated by
Graeme Chambers BA (Hons)
Medical Artist

Foreword by
David Peters MB ChB DO
Senior Lecturer, Complementary Therapy Studies
Centre for Community Care and Primary Health,
University of Westminster, London, UK

Series Editor
Professor Patrick C Pietroni FRCGP MRCP DCH
Director of the Centre for Community Care and Primary Health,
University of Westminster, London, UK

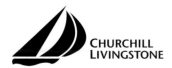
CHURCHILL
LIVINGSTONE

NEW YORK EDINBURGH LONDON MADRID MELBOURNE SAN FRANCISCO AND TOKYO 1996

CHURCHILL LIVINGSTONE
Medical Division of Pearson Professional Limited

Distributed in the United States of America by Churchill
Livingstone, 650 Avenue of the Americas, New York, N.Y.
10011, and by associated companies, branches and
representatives throughout the world.

First published 1996

ISBN 0 443 05298 0

British Library Cataloguing in Publication Data
A catalogue record for this book is available from the British
Library.

Library of Congress Cataloging in Publication Data
A catalogue record for this book is available from the
Library of Congress.

The
publisher's
policy is to use
**paper manufactured
from sustainable forests**

Produced by Longman Singapore Publishers (Pte) Ltd
Printed in Singapore

Contents

Abbreviations

AK: applied kinesiology
ATP: adenosine triphosphate
CFS: chronic fatigue syndrome
CNS: central nervous system
CSF: cerebrospinal fluid
CTM: connective tissue massage
EAV: electroacupuncture according to Voll
EMG: electromyograph
FMS: fibromyalgia syndrome
GAS: general adaptation syndrome
HSZ: hyperalgesic skin zone
INIT: integrated neuromuscular inhibition technique
LAS: local adaptation syndrome

MET: muscle energy technique/therapy (US)
MPS: myofascial pain syndrome
NGP: noxious generative points
NMT: neuromuscular technique
PNF: proprioceptive neuromuscular facilitation
PPP: periosteal pain points
PR: positional release
PSIS: posterior superior iliac spine
SCM: sternocleidomastoid
SCS: strain/counterstrain
TB: tuberculosis
TFL: tensor fascia lata
TMJ: temperomandibular joint

Foreword

This book is a *tour de force*, representing an impressive synthesis of clinical and physiological findings from diverse sources. Alongside the expected authors and researchers from osteopathy, chiropractic and musculoskeletal medicine appear references to Reich, Selye and more recent experts, such as Felix Mann and Patrick Wall.

Explanations are given of the tantalising patterns of tender and trigger points that practitioners and therapists encounter every day. The extraordinary overlapping of different systems of body mapping is both broadly reviewed and carefully analysed, with clear indications given as to how each system can be evaluated, assessed and employed in treatment settings using neuromuscular techniques (NMT).

The chapter on the varieties of reflex points alone would make the book essential reading but, in addition, there are chapters dealing with the origins of soft tissue distress and the generation of trigger and tender points. The references include names straight from the bodywork 'hall of fame': FM Alexander, Barlow, Cyriax, Feldenkrais, Karel Lewit, Vladimir Janda, Stoddard and, interestingly, Rolf; Reich, Upledger and Boadella are also included. It is good to see so erudite a work on biomechanics also cover emotional anatomy; perhaps a future edition will also examine Stanley Kellerman's work.

In explaining the why and the how of modern neuromuscular techniques, Leon Chaitow has been assisted by Judith (Walker) DeLany who has presented details of American NMT (Neuro-Muscular Therapy). What a revelation this book will be for anyone who sees osteopathy (from which the European version of neuromuscular technique evolved) as only about 'bad backs' and the manipulation of joints! Here is an outline for a whole curriculum on soft tissue work, including an important collection of ideas as to the diagnostic and therapeutic value of tender reflex points in the soft tissues of the body. The text also provides relevant therapeutic and assessment approaches relating to viscero-somatic and somatico-visceral reflexes, an area often avoided by other books. I also found the section on fibromyalgia especially useful and was particularly struck by the list differentiating it from myofascial pain syndrome.

Even well-read practitioners and therapists who use manual methods will feel as if they are taking a low-level flight over vast unknown areas of musculoskeletal literature as they read this book. I predict that almost every reader will find enlightening new avenues of knowledge and of technique which they will want to explore, and the very extensive references will help them to do so.

This book will have a long-lasting effect on the practice of many bodyworkers because Leon Chaitow has put the methods of European neuromuscular technique, originated by Stanley Lief DO and his cousin Boris Chaitow DC, into a broader context, and made NMT accessible and credible to a wide range of practitioners and therapists.

1996   D.P.

Acknowledgements

The evolution of NMT to its present position of international use would not have been possible without the work of the late Stanley Lief DO DC, his son Peter Lief DO DC and Stanley's cousin, Boris Chaitow ND DO. Boris Chaitow died, aged 87, in September 1995 during the final editing of this book. He contributed his thoughts to this text and for this, his many years of devoted clinical work and his skilled instruction, my profound thanks.

The American development of NMT owes much to the late Raymond Nimmo DC as well as to current teachers of the method, most notably Paul St. John LMT and Judith Walker LMT. Judith has produced a section of this book which outlines the particularly American variants of NMT and I wish to thank her for her time, her effort, and her skill in conveying a complex topic so well.

This book is dedicated to the memory of Stanley Lief and Boris Chaitow, and to Peter Lief, with my personal thanks for their contributions to this and other areas of health care.

1996   L.C.

Trigger points

Trigger points are localised areas of deep tenderness and increased resistance and digital pressure on such a trigger will often produce twitching and fasciculation. Pressure maintained on such a point will produce referred pain in a predictable area. If there are a number of active trigger points the reference areas may overlap.

The figure overleaf shows a selection of the most commonly found examples of representations of trigger point sites and their reference (or target) areas. Trigger points found in the same sites in different people will usually refer to the same target areas. These points are referred to throughout the text.

Sternomastoid   Splenius capitis   Temporalis   Masseter   Lower trapezius

Upper trapezius   Levator scapulae   Posterior cervical   Adductor pollicis   First interosseus

Infraspinatus   Supraspinatus   Scaleni

Iliocostalis   Multifidus   Gluteus medius

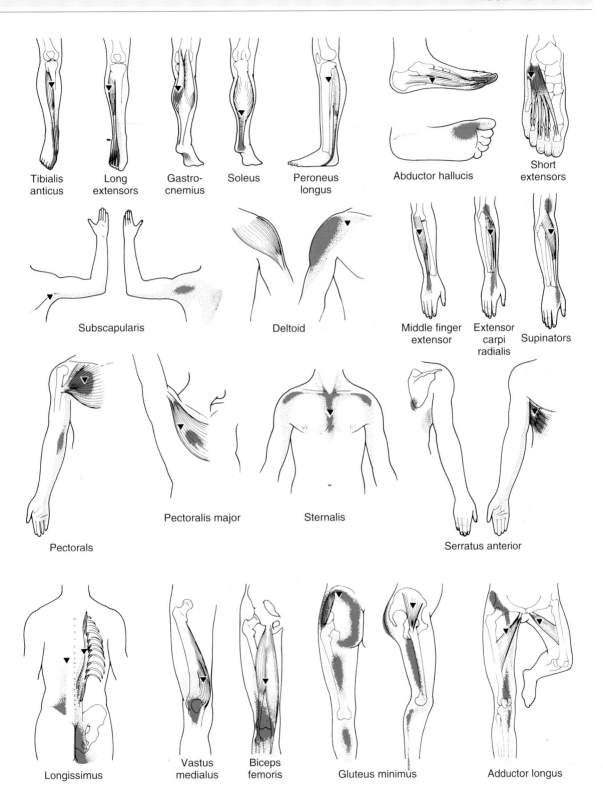

Tibialis anticus

Long extensors

Gastro-cnemius

Soleus

Peroneus longus

Abductor hallucis

Short extensors

Subscapularis

Deltoid

Middle finger extensor

Extensor carpi radialis

Supinators

Pectorals

Pectoralis major

Sternalis

Serratus anterior

Longissimus

Vastus medialus

Biceps femoris

Gluteus minimus

Adductor longus

Soft tissue distress

SOMATIC DYSFUNCTION

The musculoskeletal system is the means whereby we act out and express our human existence – 'The primary machinery of life' is what osteopathy's greatest researcher Irwin Korr (1970) called it. While, medically speaking, the musculoskeletal system may lack the glamour and fascination of vital organs and systems, the fact is that the cardiovascular and neuroendocrine and digestive (and other) systems and organs exist only to service this great machine through which we live and function. It is by means of our musculoskeletal system (not our kidneys or our livers) that we perform tasks, play games, make love, impart treatment, perform on musical instruments, paint and, in these and a multitude of other ways, interact with each other and the planet.

The musculoskeletal system is also by far the greatest energy user in the body as well as being one of our primary sources of pain, discomfort and disability, whether localised or general, referred or reflex, acute or chronic.

For the purpose of accuracy, a comprehensive term can be used to describe all lesions of the musculoskeletal system – osseous and soft tissue – and this term is 'somatic dysfunction'.

Somatic dysfunction can be defined as any impairment or altered function of related components of the somatic system (body framework) i.e. skeletal, arthrodial, and myofascial structures and related vascular, lymphatic, and neural elements. This general expression (somatic dysfunction) obviously requires specific definition in any given situation which should include identification of the particular structure, tissue or area involved.

The objectives, if not the methods we are discussing, are not new. Carl McConnell, a major force in early 20th century osteopathy, discussed the soft tissues as follows (McConnell 1962):

A pathological point of prime importance, for example, is that osseous malalignment is sustained by ligamentous rigidity. This rigidity is incepted by way of muscular fascial and tendinous tensions and stresses. Every case portrays a uniqueness in accordance with location, architectural plan and laws, tissue texture, regional and strength ratios, resident properties, environmental settings, resolution of forces etc. Remember I am speaking of the solid biological background of individual pathogenesis, the veritable soil of prediseased conditions. The lack of either sufficient, or efficient, soft-tissue work, is one reason for mediocre technique and recurrence of lesions. The same is evident in the correction of postural defects.

The causes and the results of local and general somatic dysfunction, whether traumatic, functional, postural, pathological or psychological in origin, require a brief overview as we explore different aspects of the issues and the tissues involved, so that some of their possible solutions might become apparent.

Coherent and incoherent patterns

In the next chapter we will examine one of the major causes of somatic pain and dysfunction, myofascial trigger points and the causes of this widespread phenomenon. At that time it will become clear that, while many forms of (referred) pain follow predictable and neurologically coherent pathways, there also exist patterns of pain and dysfunction which do not.

In this chapter our task is to evaluate a variety of influences on the evolution of soft tissue dysfunction, which follow a chronological sequence – the ways in which what is happening in an acute setting differs from what is taking place in a chronic situation, where an initial alarm state progressively gives way to a degree of organisation. It will also become clear that not

all muscles respond to stressors in quite the same way.

Reporting stations

The reporting mechanisms in the soft tissues and joints (Wall & Melzack 1991, Travell & Simons 1983, 1992) may be thought of as providing answers to a number of basic questions which the central nervous system requires answering.

These questions are posed by Keith Buzzell (1970) as follows: 'What is happening in the peripheral machinery with respect to three questions? What is the present position? If there is motion, where is it taking us? And, third, how fast is it taking us there?'

The various neural reporting organs provide a constant information feedback to the central nervous system and higher centres as to the current state of tone, tension, movement etc. of the tissues housing them. Such sensory information can be modulated and modified both by the influence of the mind as well as by changes in blood chemistry, to which the sympathetic nervous system is sensitive. A variety of inputs of information will give the answers to these important questions which allow the body to provide appropriate responses to the demands and adaptations constantly called for by varying situations. Some important structures involved in this internal information highway are:

Ruffini end-organs. These are found within the joint capsule, around the joint, so that each is responsible for describing what is happening over an angle of approximately 15°, with a degree of overlap between it and the adjacent end-organ. These are not easily fatigued organs, and are progressively recruited as the joint moves, so that movement is smooth and not jerky. The prime concern of Ruffini end-organs is to maintain a steady position. They are also, to some extent, concerned with reporting the direction of movement.

Golgi end-organs. These, too, adapt slowly, and continue to discharge over a lengthy period. They are found in the ligaments associated with the joint. Unlike the Ruffini end-organs, which respond to muscular contraction which alters tension in the joint capsule, Golgi end-organs are not thus affected, and can deliver information independently of the state of muscular contraction. This helps the body to know just where the joint is at any given moment, irrespective of muscular activity.

The Pacinian corpuscle. This is found in periarticular connective tissue, and adapts rapidly. It triggers discharges, and then ceases reporting in a very short space of time. These messages occur successively, during motion, and the CNS can therefore be aware of the rate of acceleration of movement taking place in the area. It is sometimes called an acceleration receptor.

There are other end-organs, but these three can be seen to provide information as to the present position, direction and rate of movement of any joint.

Muscle spindle. This receptor is sensitive and complex. It detects, evaluates, reports and adjusts the length of the muscle in which it lies, setting its tone. Acting with the Golgi tendon organ, most of the information as to muscle tone and movement is reported. The spindles lie parallel to the muscle fibres, and are attached to either skeletal muscle, or the tendinous portion of the muscle. Inside the spindle are fibres which may be one of two types. One is described as a 'nuclear bag' fibre, and the other as a chain fibre. In different muscles the ratios of these internal spindle fibres differ. In the centre of the spindle is a receptor called the annulospiral receptor (or primary ending) and on each side of this lies a 'flower spray receptor' (secondary ending). The primary ending discharges rapidly, and this occurs in response to even small changes in muscle length. The secondary ending compensates for this, because it fires messages only when larger changes in muscle length have occurred.

The spindle is a 'length comparator', and it may discharge for long periods at a time. Within the spindle there are fine, intrafusal fibres which alter the sensitivity of the spindle. These can be altered without any actual change taking place in the length of the muscle itself, via an independent gamma efferent supply to the intrafusal fibres. This has implications in a variety of acute and chronic problems.

Buzzell (1970) describes the neural connections with the CNS thus:

The central connections of the spindle receptors are important. The annulospiral fibre has the only known monosynaptic relationship in the body. As the fibre passes to the cord, and through the dorsal horn, it goes without synapse, directly to the anterior horn cells that serve the muscle fibres in the vicinity of the spindle. This is the basis of the so called 'tendon reflex', which actually is not a tendon reflex, but simply a spindle response to a sudden elongation of the muscle.

In contrast, the secondary fibres have various synapses in their central connection which can be traced to higher cortical centres. Conscious activity may therefore provide a modifying influence, via these structures, on muscle tone. The activities of the spindle appear to provide information as to length, velocity of contraction and changes in velocity. How long is the muscle? How quickly is it changing length? And what is happening to this rate of change of length? (Gray 1977)

Golgi tendon receptors. These structures indicate how hard the muscle is working since they reflect the tension of the muscle, rather than its length, as does the spindle. If the tendon organ detects excessive overload it may cause cessation of function of the muscle, to prevent damage. This produces relaxation.

There exist various ways of 'manipulating' the neural reporting stations to produce physiological modifications in soft tissues – notably of the Golgi tendon organ in muscle energy techniques (MET) and of the spindle in various positional release (PR) techniques, such as strain/counterstrain (SCS). (Jones 1980, Stiles 1984)

Effect of contradictory information

Korr's words regarding the nature of the information which these, and other, reporting stations are providing to the CNS are worth recording (Korr 1976). He reminds us:

The spinal cord is the keyboard on which the brain plays when it calls for activity or for change in activity. But each 'key' in the console sounds, not an individual 'tone', such as the contraction of a particular group of muscle fibres, but a whole 'melody' of activity, even a 'symphony' of motion. In other words, built into the cord is a large repertoire of patterns of activity, each involving the complex, harmonious, delicately balanced orchestration of the contractions and relaxations of many muscles. The brain 'thinks' in terms of whole motions, not individual muscles. It calls selectively, for the preprogrammed patterns in the cord and brain stem, modifying them in countless ways and combining them in an infinite variety of still more complex patterns. Each activity is also subject to further modulation, refinement, and adjustment by the afferent feedback continually streaming in from the participating muscles, tendons, and joints.

This means that the pattern of information fed back to the CNS and brain reflects, at any given time, the steady state of joints, the direction as well as speed of alteration in position of joints, together with data on the length of muscle fibres, the degree of load that is being borne, along with the tension this involves. This total input is what occurs, rather than individual pieces of information, as outlined above, from particular reporting stations. But what if any of the mass of information being constantly received should be contradictory, and actually conflict with the other information being received?

Buzzell puts it this way:

It is possible, for example, for the excessive force exerted by external trauma to induce such hyperactivity of the joint and muscle receptors that the reports from that area become gibberish.

Should conflicting reports reach the cord from a variety of sources simultaneously, no discernible pattern may be recognised by the CNS. In such a case no adequate response would be forthcoming, and it is probable that activity would be stopped. Spasm, or splinting could therefore result.

Korr (1976) discusses a variety of insults which may result in increased neural excitability: the triggering of a barrage of *supernumerary* impulses, to and from the cord, and also what he terms 'cross-talk', in which axons may overload and pass impulses to one another directly; muscle contraction disturbances, vasomotion, pain impulses, reflex mechanisms, disturbances in sym-

pathetic activity, all may result from such activity, due to what might be relatively slight tissue changes, for example, in the intervertebral foramina.

In addition, Korr states that when any tissue is disturbed, whether bone, joint, ligament or muscle, the local stresses feed constant information to the cord, and effectively jam normal patterned transmission from the periphery. These factors, combined with any mechanical alterations in the tissues, are the background to much somatic dysfunction. He summarises thus:

These are the somatic insults, the sources of incoherent, and meaningless feedback, that causes the spinal cord to halt normal operations and to freeze the status quo in the offending and offended tissues. It is these phenomena that are detectable at the body surface, and are reflected in disorders of muscle tension, tissue texture, visceral and circulatory function, and even secretory function; the elements that are so much a part of osteopathic diagnosis.

Trophic neural influences

Setting aside for the moment the obviously important feature of nerves and their message-carrying functions we need to consider the less understood role they play in transporting substances – proteins, phospholipids, glycoproteins, neurotransmitters, enzymes, mitochondria and more. Transportation takes place, at a rate of anything from 1 mm/24 h to several hundred mm/24 h depending upon what is being transported and the presence, or not, of interfering factors (see below, p. 7). Movement occurs in both directions along nerves, with retrograde (returning from the target tissues towards the central nervous system) transportation seemingly 'a fundamental means of communication between neurons and between neurons and non-neuronal cells' which strongly influences the 'plasticity of the nervous system' according to Korr's research (Korr 1981).

Korr has once again set the scene for us via his diligent research over half a century, when he describes just how vulnerable these highways of nutrition are: 'Any factor which causes derangement of transport mechanisms in the axon, or that chronically alters the quality or quantity of the axonally transported substances, could cause the trophic influences to become detrimental. This alteration in turn would produce aberrations of structure, function and metabolism, thereby contributing to dysfunction and disease.'

And what can cause such neurotrophic interference? Korr specifies, 'Deformations of nerves and roots, such as compression, stretching, angulation and torsion,' especially, he tells us, 'in their passage over highly mobile joints, through bony canals, intervertebral foramina, fascial layers and tonically contracted muscles.'

Butler's contribution

Physiotherapist David Butler (1991) has shown how adverse tension in the nervous system can impair its mobility and elasticity and how many painful problems can result from this factor. His detailed analysis of the diagnosis and treatment of such restrictions and tensions is highly recommended to manual therapists.

NMT'S ROLE

Our task in understanding, assessing and dealing with this complex of somatic dysfunction is aided by the diagnostic and therapeutic ability of neuromuscular technique, as well as by the more recent development of muscle energy and 'positional release' techniques, all of which we may employ in attempting to normalise dysfunctional soft tissue states. In order to understand the context for application of such approaches we need to appreciate the influence of time on such changes.

General adaptation syndrome (GAS) and local adaptation syndrome (LAS) – and connective tissue

Selye (1976) called stress the non-specific element in disease production. In describing the relationship between the general adaptation syndrome (GAS) – i.e. alarm reaction, resistance (adaptation) phase followed by the exhaustion phase (when adaptation finally fails) which affects the organism as a whole – and the local adaptation

syndrome (LAS) which affects a specific stressed area of the body, Selye emphasised the importance of connective tissue. He demonstrated that stress results in a pattern of adaptation, individual to each organism. He also showed that, when an individual is acutely alarmed, stressed, aroused, homeostatic (self-normalising) mechanisms are activated – this is the alarm reaction of Selye's general adaptation syndrome and local adaptation syndrome.

If the alarm status is prolonged or repetitive, defensive adaptation processes commence and produce long-term, chronic, changes. In assessing, palpating, the patient these neuro-musculoskeletal changes represent a record of the attempts on the part of the body to adapt and adjust to the stresses imposed upon it as time passes. The results of repeated postural and traumatic insults of a lifetime, combined with changes of emotional and psychological origin, will often present a confusing pattern of tense, contracted, bunched, fatigued and ultimately fibrous tissue (Chaitow 1989).

The minutiae of the process are not for the moment at issue. What is important is the realisation that, due to prolonged stress of a postural, psychic or mechanical type, discrete areas of the body become so altered by the efforts to compensate and adapt, that structural and, eventually, pathological changes become apparent. Researchers have shown that the type of stress involved can be entirely physical in nature (Wall & Melzack 1989) (e.g. a single injury or repetitive postural strain) or purely psychic in nature (Latey 1983) (e.g. chronically repressed anger). More often than not, though, a combination of emotional and physical stresses will so alter neuro-musculo-skeletal structures as to create a series of identifiable physical changes, which will themselves generate further stress, such as pain, joint restriction, general discomfort and fatigue.

Predictable chain reactions of compensating changes will evolve in the soft tissues in most instances of chronic adaptation to biomechanical and psychogenic stress (Lewit 1992). Such adaptation will be seen to be almost always at the expense of optimum function, as well as being an ongoing source of further physiological embarrassment.

The aim of this book is to emphasise the importance of the soft tissues in such dysfunction and to explain the use of one particular assessment and therapeutic tool – neuromuscular technique.

Stress response sequence
(Basmajian 1974, Dvorak & Dvorak 1984, Janda 1982, Janda 1983, Korr 1978, Lewit 1985, Travell & Simons 1983/1992)

When the musculoskeletal system is 'stressed' a sequence of events occurs which can be summarised as follows:

- 'Something' (see Causes of soft tissue dysfunction below, p. 7) occurs which leads to increased muscular tone.
- Increased tone, if anything but short-term, leads to a retention of metabolic wastes.
- Increased tone simultaneously leads to a degree of localised oxygen lack (relative to the efforts being demanded of the tissues) – resulting in ischaemia.
- Increased tone might also lead to a degree of oedema.
- These factors (retention of wastes/ischaemia/oedema) result in discomfort/pain.
- Discomfort/pain leads to increased or maintained hypertonicity.
- Inflammation, or at least chronic irritation, may be a result.
- Neurological reporting stations in hypertonic tissues will bombard the CNS with information regarding their status, leading to a degree of sensitisation of neural structures and the evolution of facilitation – hyper-reactivity (see Ch. 2).
- Macrophages are activated, as is increased vascularity and fibroblastic activity.
- Connective tissue production increases with cross linkage leading to shortened fascia.
- Since all fascia/connective tissue is continuous throughout the body any distortions which develop in one region can potentially create distortions elsewhere, so negatively influencing structures which are supported by, or

attached to the fascia, including nerves, muscles, lymph structures and blood vessels.
- Changes occur in the elastic (muscle) tissues, leading to chronic hypertonicity and, ultimately, to fibrotic changes.
- Hypertonicity in a muscle will produce inhibition of its antagonist muscles.
- Chain reactions evolve in which some muscles (postural – Type I) shorten, while others (phasic – Type II) weaken.
- Because of sustained increased muscle tension, ischaemia in tendinous structures occurs, as it does in localised areas of muscles. Periosteal pain areas develop.
- Abnormal biomechanics occurs, involving malcoordination of movement (with antagonist muscle groups being hypertonic – for example erector spinae – and weak – for example weak rectus abdominis group).
- Joint restrictions and/or imbalances as well as fascial shortenings develop.
- Progressive evolution of localised areas of hyper-reactivity of neural structures occurs (facilitated areas) in paraspinal regions or within muscles (trigger points).
- The degree of energy wastage due to unnecessarily maintained hypertonicity leads to generalised fatigue.
- More widespread functional changes develop – for example affecting respiratory function – with repercussions on the total economy of the body.
- In the presence of a constant neurological feedback of impulses to the CNS/brain from neural reporting stations indicating heightened arousal (a hypertonic muscle status is the alarm reaction of the flight/fight alarm response) there will be increased levels of psychological arousal and an inability to relax adequately with consequent increase in hypertonicity.
- Functional patterns of use of a biologically unsustainable nature will emerge, probably involving chronic musculoskeletal problems and pain.
- At this stage, restoration of normal function requires therapeutic input which addresses the multiple changes which have occurred as

well as the need to re-educate the individual as to how to use their body, to breathe, to carry and to use themselves in less stressful ways.

- The chronic adaptive changes which develop in such a scenario lead to the increased likelihood of future acute exacerbations as the progressively chronic less supple and resilient biomechanical structures attempt to cope with new stress factors resulting from the normal demands of modern living.

CAUSES OF SOFT TISSUE DYSFUNCTION

The 'something' which can contribute to the sequence described above (Stress response sequence, p. 6) includes:

- Congenital factors (short/long leg, small hemipelvis, fascial, cranial and other distortions)
- Overuse, misuse and abuse (and disuse) factors (such as injury or inappropriate patterns of use involved in work, sport or regular activities)
- Postural stresses
- Chronic negative emotional states (anxiety etc.)
- Reflexive factors (trigger points, facilitated spinal regions).

As a result of the processes described above – which affect each and every one of us to some degree – acute and painful problems overlaid on chronic soft tissue changes become the norm – the raw material on which bodywork therapies focus.

Stressing the soft tissues

Forms of stress affecting the body can be categorised as follows – physiological, emotional, behavioural and structural (Barlow 1959).

Physiological. This might involve an overall increase of muscle hypertonicity/tension or localised soft tissue changes due to habitual patterns of use or from patterns of overuse. Occupational, sporting, leisure and general activities are all potential producers of such

repetitive or constant stress involving the soft tissues (Janda 1988, Lewit 1993).

Emotional. All emotional changes are mirrored in muscular changes. Emotional attitudes such as anger or fear, as well as moods such as excitement, anxiety or depression, are known to produce altered muscular postures and patterns. There is a close relationship between habitual tension patterns and posture, and psychological attitudes and conflicts. The use of the body as a metaphor for emotional feelings ('pain in the neck') is well documented (Boadella 1978).

Reich (1949) outlined his understanding of the postures and defensive armouring produced by neurotic patients. He believed that such individuals often behaved as though they were 'half-dead' and that their normal functioning, on all levels, was diminished and restricted. He describes an all too frequently seen pattern: 'They were disturbed sexually, they were disturbed in their work function, their bodily processes lacked rhythm, their breathing was uncoordinated' (Boadella 1978).

Reich and his followers demonstrated how emotions can 'mobilise' or 'paralyse' the body, with continued and repeated stress producing 'blockages' and restrictions which, if unreleased, become self-perpetuating and are themselves the source of pain and further stress. The ability to relax is lost, and the drain on nervous energy is profound in such situations.

The bioenergetic answer to this problem is to aid in the release of these tensions by a complex set of exercises, including facial expressions and body positions, accompanied by breathing techniques. These methods are doubtless successful in many cases, but what concerns our present study is recognition that neuromuscular changes, as evidenced by stiffness, pain and restriction, may often be a manifestation of deep psychological and emotional stress.

Behavioural. All movement requires muscular activity. Certain patterns of use establish themselves. Often, individual awareness of the pattern of use is diminished, and habitually used repetitive actions take place with resultant muscular hypertonicity developing (Feldenkrais 1977). Altering habitual use patterns is far more difficult than altering the resultant soft tissue changes short-term. Breathing patterns which are habitual, such as hyperventilation, could be included in this category of stress factors impacting the musculoskeletal system.

Structural. Over and above inborn features, such as a short leg, acquired structural changes make further demands on the adaptive capacity of the body. Depending upon the mechanical and structural loads it bears and responds to, muscle tissue will change in texture, chemistry, tone etc. and will also modify and alter the framework of the body, warping and cramping its potential for normal use. The body will be bent and distorted to meet the stresses imposed from without and within.

Barlow, whose work follows that of Alexander (1957), suggests that there exists a self-regulating tendency in the way muscles behave in response to stress. The term 'postural homeostasis' implies a return to a balanced resting state after activity. Such regulation is usually at an unconscious level and he gives the example of a patient with persistent low back pain who, in the resting position, demonstrates a particular set of muscular distortions such as tense erector spina muscles on the left and a tense trapezius on the right, together with a pelvic twist to the right. On activity all these spasms would become accentuated. Barlow employed postural re-education (Alexander Technique) to restore balanced use; however, it is suggested that more long-lasting benefits might be achieved by the use of soft tissue normalisation, using NMT, muscle energy and myofascial release methods, plus appropriate manipulation – combined with re-education – rather than simply relying on re-education without attention to the structural modifications (fibrosis for example) which the adaptation process had produced. Any attempt to normalise structural changes without due attention to patterns of use would be equally unsatisfactory.

Source of pain

Where pain exists in tense musculature, Barlow suggests that in the absence of other pathology such pain results from:

1. The muscle itself, through some noxious metabolic product (this has been called 'Factor P' (Lewis 1942)), or an interference in blood circulation due to spasm, resulting in relative ischaemia.

2. The muscular insertion into the periosteum, such as that caused by an actual lifting of the periosteal tissue following marked, or repetitive, muscular tension (e.g. 'tennis elbow' and periosteal pain points which are described and listed in Chapter 3). (Lewit 1993)

3. The joint, which can become restricted and over-approximated. In advanced cases, osteoarthritic changes can result from the regular microtrauma of repeated muscular misuse. Over-approximation of joint surfaces due to soft tissue shortening can also lead to uneven wear and tear, as for example when the tensor fascia lata structure shortens and crowds both the hip and lateral knee joint structures.

4. Nerve irritation, which can be produced spinally or along the course of the nerve as a result of chronic muscular contractions. These can involve disc and general spinal mechanical faults (Korr 1976).

5. Variations in pain threshold, largely to do with perception (Melzack 1983), which will make all these factors more or less significant and obvious.

Baldry (1993) describes the progression from muscle in a normal state to one in painful chronic distress, as commonly involving initial or repetitive trauma (strain or excessive use) resulting in the release of chemical substances such as bradykinin, prostaglandins, histamine, serotonin and potassium ions. Sensitisation of A-delta and C (Group IV) sensory nerve fibres may follow with involvement of the brain (limbic system and the frontal lobe).

Trigger points (see Ch. 3) which evolve from such a progression, themselves become the source of new problems in their own locality, as well as at distant sites, as their sarcoplasmic reticulum is damaged and free calcium ions are released, leading to the formation of localised taut bands of tissue (involving the actin–myosin contractile mechanisms in the muscle sarcomeres). If free calcium and energy-producing ATP is present this becomes a self-perpetuating feature compounded by the relative (to surrounding tissues) ischaemia which has been identified in such chronically contracted tissues (Simons 1987). Local myofascial changes are considered in Chapter 3 (p. 35).

Where pain has been produced by repetitive habits, postural and otherwise, with emotional and psychological overtones, the task of the therapist is complex since hypertonicity can often only be partially released or relaxed without resolving the underlying pattern of use. If repeated recurrence of painful episodes is to be minimised, a state of relative equilibrium of body structure and function is needed which calls for both treatment of structural restrictions as well as re-education as to posture and use.

Stoddard, in discussing contracted musculature (Stoddard 1969), describes its 'stringy' feel, resulting from the continuous contraction of some muscle fibres and ascribes the cause to the underlying joint dysfunctions. The resulting ache and pain, he believes, is usually a result of circulatory embarrassment as metabolic wastes build up due to sustained muscular contraction. Muscular guarding is always seen to indicate deeper pathological changes (e.g. TB of the spine, osteomyelitis, disc herniation etc.).

Stoddard sees the metabolic wastes, which may result from a degree of stasis, as causing a vicious cycle in perpetuating muscular contraction, leading eventually to fibrous changes occurring. There is no indication that Stoddard considers such changes to be of primary importance in his treatment programme. He does stress the importance of exercises, to strengthen muscle groups, and of correct posture, but does not indicate any great interest in treatment of the soft tissues themselves.

While release of muscular restrictions and shortening could be seen to be a desirable step in the restoration of normality, it is worth emphasising that once adaptive, fibrotic changes have taken place in the soft tissues (whether in response to emotional stress or anything else) these changes are no longer under purely neurological control and therefore cannot simply be 'released' (by exercises or anything else) but require a physical input which alters, stretches

and effectively breaks down concretions such as fibrotic tissue.

Different responses in postural and phasic muscles
(Engel et al 1986, Woo et al 1987)

It is not within the scope of this book to provide detailed physiological analysis; however, it is vital that the ways in which different muscle fibre types respond to stress are understood.

Muscles have a mixture of fibre types, although in most there is a predominance of one sort or another. There are those which contract slowly ('slow twitch fibres' or 'slow white fibres') which are classified as Type I. These have very low stores of energy-supplying glycogen but carry high concentrations of myoglobulin and mitochondria. These fibres fatigue slowly and are mainly involved in postural and stabilising tasks.

There are also several phasic/active Type II fibre forms, notably:

- Type IIa fibres ('fast twitch' or 'fast red' fibres) which contract more speedily than Type I, and are moderately resistant to fatigue with relatively high concentrations of mitochondria and myoglobulin.
- Type IIb fibres ('fast twitch/glycolytic fibres' or 'fast white fibres') which are less fatigue-resistant and depend more on glycolytic sources of energy, with low levels of mitochondria and myoglobulin.
- Type IIm ('superfast' fibre) found mainly in the jaw muscles which depend upon a unique myosin structure which, along with a high glycogen content, differentiates it from the other Type II fibres (Rowlerson 1981).

The implications of the effects of prolonged stress on these different muscle types cannot be too strongly emphasised, since long-term stress involving Type I muscles indicates that they will shorten, whereas Type II fibres – undergoing similar stress – will weaken without shortening over their whole length (they may however develop shortened areas within the muscle). It is important to emphasise that shortness/tightness of a postural muscle does not imply strength. Such muscles may test as strong or weak.

However, a weak phasic muscle will not shorten overall and will always test as weak.

Fibre type is not totally fixed, in that evidence exists as to the potential for adaptability of muscles, so that committed muscle fibres can be transformed from slow-twitch to fast-twitch and vice versa (Lin 1994).

An example of this potential, which is of profound clinical significance, involves the scalene muscles which Lewit confirms can be classified as either postural or phasic (Lewit 1985). If the largely phasic, dedicated to movement, scalene muscles have postural functions thrust upon them (as in an asthmatic condition in which they will attempt to maintain the upper ribs in elevation so as to enhance lung capacity) and if, due to the laboured breathing of such an individual, they are thoroughly and regularly stressed, their fibre type will alter and they will shorten – becoming postural muscles.

The muscles' role in low back pain problems

If we examine the role of the muscular component of the musculoskeletal structures we find strong evidence as to its involvement in many acute and chronic conditions. Jokl (1984) tells us that disuse muscular atrophy, following back injury, is a major factor in the progression from an acute back problem to a chronic one. Changes take place which are observable, histologically and biochemically, in the muscle fibres, and which are translated into functional changes. The effects of these changes involves decreased endurance and weakened muscles, as well as spasm. We should remind ourselves of the basic anatomy of the low back, which includes the division of the musculature into :

1. The *deep muscles*, connecting the adjacent spinous processes (interspinales), adjacent transverse processes (intertransversari) and the rotatores, connecting the transverse process below to the laminae above.

2. The *intermediate muscles* include multifidus, which connects the transverse processes to the spinous processes of the vertebra above.

3. The *superficial group* includes iliocostalis, longissimus and spinalis (erector spinae). The

origin of this is on the ischium, and the insertion on the 6th and 12th ribs. Together with the psoas, major and minor, and the quadratus, these greatly influence spinal stability.

4. The *prevertebral muscles*, which further stabilise and support the spine, are those which encircle the abdomen, such as the internal and external oblique, and rectus abdominus muscles.

MUSCLE TYPES

Any, or all, of these muscles can have a major influence of the onset of low back problems and pain. The division of muscles relating to their different postural and phasic (volitional movement) types is worthy of re-emphasis. As mentioned above (p. 9) muscle fibres may be differentiated into types by virtue of their role, as well as their main energy source. For example, Type I muscles require stamina, rather than speed of action, and derive their energy via oxidative phosphorylation. This is in contrast to Type II muscles which produce power and speed and derive energy from carbohydrate sources via glycolytic breakdown.

The muscles which support the spine are mainly Type I, endurance and stamina muscles. Their activities are in the main related to static, anti-gravity efforts, which require prolonged contraction and these muscles are far more susceptible to disuse atrophy and shortening. The strength of such muscles may not indicate much change, even after a period of disuse, but the endurance factor could be greatly affected. This makes for a certain degree of caution being required in interpreting muscle strength tests involving the paravertebral musculature.

Jokl points out that EMG studies indicate that paraspinal muscles show marked fatigue in individuals with low back pain. This fatigue factor may play a major part in worsening, or accentuating, an already demonstrable degree of dysfunction in such a region. When such a situation exists (pain and easy fatigue of supporting musculature) it may be assumed that an increasing number of muscle fibres have been recruited in order to maintain spinal stability, which in turn results in increased muscular pressure. Jokl tells us that normal muscle can work for long periods without any EMG evidence of fatigue. As muscles become weaker, they work at an increased percentage of their maximum voluntary contraction. Ultimately this leads to muscle spasm, which allows ischaemia to develop, and pain to result.

The cycle of increased effort, local spasm and ischaemia, leading to pain, may ultimately result in paraspinal spasm and splinting.

The use of both neuromuscular technique and muscle energy techniques is indicated in such a situation, as a means of breaking the cycle and, initially, relaxing the contracted muscles. NMT methods have a combined effect, both relaxing the tissues as well as increasing the vascularity and mobility of these structures. They become more 'extensible', to use Grieve's phrase (Grieve 1985).

He enlarges on this aspect thus:

There is new evidence to support the view that suppleness and flexibility of muscle and connective tissue, are of prime importance. Long and continued occupational and postural stress, asymmetrically imposed upon the soft tissues, tends to cause fibroblasts to multiply more rapidly and produce more collagen. Besides occupying more space within the connective tissue element of the muscle, the extra fibres encroach on the space normally occupied by nerves and vessels. Because of this trespass, the tissue loses elasticity and may become painful when the muscle is required to do work in coordination with others. In the long term collagen would replace the active fibres of the muscle and since collagen is fairly resistant to enzyme breakdown these changes tend to be irreversible.

Jokl, Korr, Patterson and Grieve help us to gain a clearer picture of the structural changes taking place as stress factors operating over a period of time impact on the soft tissues.

Postural and phasic muscle lists

Thus Type I postural muscles are prone to loss of endurance capabilities when disused or subject to pathological influences and become shortened or tighter, while Type II phasic muscles, when abused or disused, become weak.

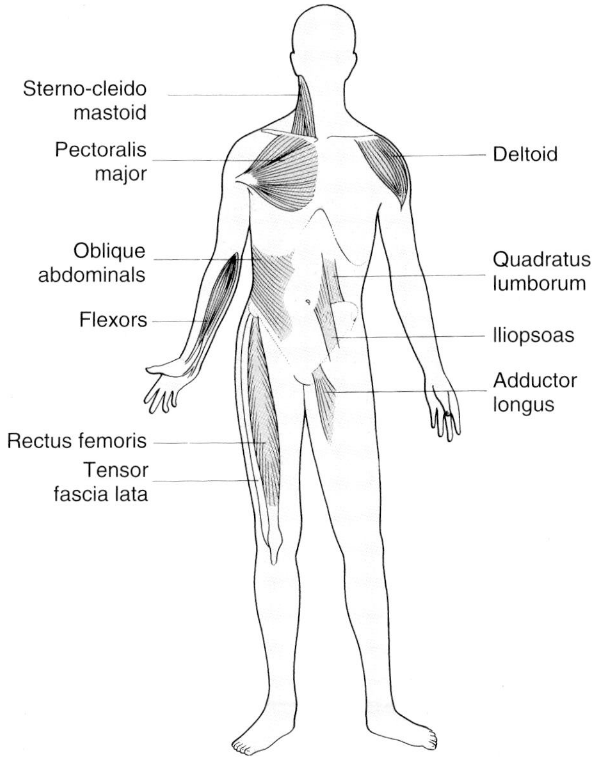

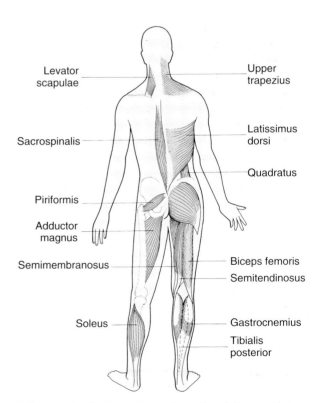

Figure 1.1A The major postural muscles of the anterior aspect of the body.

Figure 1.1B The major postural muscles of the posterior aspect of the body.

Among the more important postural muscles which become hypertonic in response to dysfunction are (Fig. 1.1):

- Trapezius (upper), sternocleidomastoid, levator scapulae and upper aspects of pectoralis major, in the upper trunk; and the flexors of the arms.
- Quadratus lumborum, erector spinae, oblique abdominals and iliopsoas, in the lower trunk.
- Tensor fascia lata, rectus femoris, biceps femoris, adductors (longus brevis and magnus) piriformis, hamstrings, semitendinosus, in the pelvic and lower extremity region.

Phasic muscles, which weaken in response to dysfunction (i.e. are inhibited) include:

- The paravertebral muscles (not erector spinae) and scaleni, the extensors of the upper extremity (flexors are primarily postural) the abdominal aspects of pectoralis major; middle and inferior aspects of trapezium; the rhomboids, serratus anterior, rectus abdominus; the internal and external obliques, gluteals, the peroneal muscles and the extensors of the arms.
- Muscle groups such as the scaleni are equivocal – they start out as phasic muscles but can end up as postural ones (see above, p. 10).[1]

Fibrositis

Having evolved from 'muscular rheumatism', via fibrositis to the currently favoured term 'fibromyalgia', generalised muscular pain is a manifestation of multiple causative influences.

The great British orthopaedic physician and writer James Cyriax (1962) believed, like Stoddard, that all primary 'fibrositic' conditions were a result of articular lesions (dysfunctions). A secondary fibrositic change could result, he

stated, from traumatic injury to soft tissues (e.g. capsular adhesion at the shoulder after injury) which he called fibrosis, not fibrositis. He saw fibrosis as scar tissue formation. Other secondary fibrositic conditions were said to result from rheumatoid disease, infection (such as epidemic myalgia) and parasitic infection (*triclina spiralis*). All other muscular and soft tissue dysfunctions, Cyriax regarded as one result of joint dysfunction which then produced muscular protective spasm, muscular wasting, pain etc., and which could only be normalised by correction of the joint lesion.

NMT theory and practice holds an almost precisely opposite view to that held by Cyriax – maintaining that appropriate normalisation of the soft tissues can, more often than not, achieve joint normalisation when restriction exists, without active manipulation of the joint, since most joint problems appear to be the direct result of myofascial dysfunction (Cantu & Grodin 1992, Janda 1988, Stiles 1984).

Cyriax did point out that fibrous tissue is capable of maintaining inflammation, originally traumatic, almost as a matter of habit. In such cases he opted for hydrocortisone injections as the appropriate measure to 'break' this habit. Such treatment can work, but such an approach all too often fails if underlying fibrotic changes have not been normalised or habits of use modified.

Fibrositis changes its name to fibromyalgia

In Chapter 3, in which the phenomenon of local soft tissue dysfunction, most notably myofascial trigger point activity, is analysed in detail, the evolution of thinking regarding 'fibrositis' is also examined. Fibromyalgia (the new incarnation of fibrositis) with its causes, associated conditions and diagnostic criteria require discussion in that context because of the confusion which currently exists as to the overlap between fibromyalgia syndrome (FMS), myofascial pain syndrome (MPS) and chronic fatigue syndrome (CFS). The fascia of the body has profound influence, and it is to this focus which we now turn.

---

[1]Lewit (1985) does not subscribe to the theory that phasic and postural muscles can be differentiated by virtue of their fibre type, as do Grieve and Jokl, but certainly subscribes to their differences in all other regards.

THE FASCIAL NETWORK
(DiGiovanna 1991, Frankel 1980, Warwick & Williams 1973)

Of major significance in understanding musculo-skeletal function and dysfunction is the fact that the fascia comprises one connected network – from the fascia attached to the inner aspects of the skull to the fascia in the soles of the feet there exists just one fascial structure. If any part of this is deformed or distorted there may be negative stresses imposed on distant aspects – and on the structures which it divides, envelops, enmeshes, and supports and with which it connects. There is ample evidence that Wolff's Law applies, in that fascia accommodates to chronic stress patterns and deforms itself – something which often precedes deformity of osseous and cartilaginous structures in chronic diseases.

The musculoskeletal system, the mechanical component of the human machine, comprising as it does 60% of the mass of the body, exists in a state of structural and functional continuity between all of its hard and soft tissues. And it is the connective tissues/fascia which provide most of that continuity. Any tendency to think of a local 'lesion' as existing in isolation should be discouraged as we try to visualise a complex, interrelated, symbiotically functioning assort-ment of tissues comprising skin, muscles, liga-ments, tendons and bones, as well as the neural structures, blood and lymph channels and vessels which bisect and invest these tissues – all given shape, cohesion and functional ability by the fascia (connective tissue).

Apart from its immense role in the support, structural organisation and motion of the body, fascia is involved in numerous complex bio-chemical activities:

• Connective tissue provides a supporting matrix for more highly organised structures and attaches extensively to muscles. Individ-ual muscle fibres are enveloped by endo-mysium, which is connected to the stronger perimysium which surrounds the fasciculi. The perimysium's fibres attach to the even stronger epimysium, which surrounds the muscle as a whole and which attaches to fascial tissues nearby.

• Because it contains mesenchymal cells of an embryonic type, connective tissue provides a generalised tissue capable of giving rise, under certain circumstances, to more specialised elements.

• It provides, by its fascial planes, pathways for nerves, blood and lymphatic vessels and structures.

• Many of the neural structures in fascia are sensory in nature.

• It supplies restraining mechanisms by the dif-ferentiation of retention bands, fibrous pulleys and check ligaments, as well as assisting in the harmonious production and control of movement.

• Where connective tissue is loose in texture it allows movement between adjacent struc-tures and, by the formation of bursal sacs, it reduces the effects of pressure and friction.

• Deep fascia ensheaths and preserves the characteristic contour of the limbs, and promotes the circulation in the veins and lymphatic vessels.

• The superficial fascia, which forms the pan-niculus adiposus, allows for the storage of fat and also provides a surface covering which aids in the conservation of body heat.

• By virtue of its fibroblastic activity, connec-tive tissue aids in the repair of injuries by the deposition of collagenous fibres (scar tissue).

• The ensheathing layer of deep fascia, as well as intermuscular septa and interosseous mem-branes, provides vast surface areas used for muscular attachment.

• The meshes of loose connective tissue contain the 'tissue fluid' and provide an essential medium through which the cellular elements of other tissues are brought into functional relation with blood and lymph. Connective tissue has a nutritive function and houses nearly a quarter of all body fluids (Dicke 1978).

• The histiocytes of connective tissue comprise part of an important defence mechanism against bacterial invasion by their phagocytic activity. They also play a part as scavengers in removing cell debris and foreign material.

- Connective tissue represents an important 'neutraliser' or detoxicator to both endogenous toxins (those produced under physiological conditions), and exogenous toxins (those which are introduced from outside the organism). The mechanical barrier presented by connective tissue has important defensive functions in cases of infection and toxaemia.

Fascia, then, is not just a background structure with little function apart from its obvious supporting role, but is an ubiquitous, tenacious, connective tissue which is deeply involved in almost all of the fundamental processes of the body's structure, function and metabolism.

In therapeutic terms there can be little logic in trying to consider muscle as a separate structure from fascia since they are so intimately related. Remove connective tissue from the scene and any muscle left would be a jelly-like structure without form or functional ability.

Soft tissue changes – energy and fascial considerations

Taylor (1958) has postulated that tissue changes, apparent to the trained palpating hand, often result from changes in thermodynamic equilibrium. He states that the body is a thermodynamic system and, as such, the alterations in the extracellular fluids, viscosity, pH, electrophoretic changes, colloidal osmotic pressure, etc. are subject to thermodynamic laws. One of these laws states that the total energy of such a system and its surroundings must remain constant, though the energy may be changed from one form to another due to alterations of the stresses imposed.

For example, through postural stress and gravitational effects, particular changes in the fascia involved would result in energy loss and therefore stasis and stagnation. One of the characteristics of thermodynamics is that of thixotropy, in which gels become more solid with energy loss and more fluid with energy input. Such changes are certainly palpable in soft tissues before and after neuromuscular and other forms of manual treatment. Taylor has stated that manipulative pressure and stretching are the most effective ways of modifying energy potentials of abnormal soft tissues.

Little (1969) believes that an additional beneficial effect results from the interaction of the bioenergy mechanism of the practitioner and the bioenergy field of the patient.

Eeman (1947) has shown that after each simple movement that we perform we retain a degree of unconscious contractile muscular activity. This unconscious continuation of objective contraction is not only wasteful of energy but productive of long-term changes within the tissues involved. He has also shown that unless, and until, neuromuscular relaxation is achieved there cannot be a total resting state of the mind.

Over and above the important factors of posture, functional ability and pain, the musculoskeletal component of the body plays a vital role in the conservation – wastage – of energy and in the attainment, or otherwise, of a truly relaxed mind. Whilst the origins of musculoskeletal dysfunction can be either psychic or physical, the constant interaction of the soma with the mind ensures a degree of psychic stress occurring as a feedback from physically caused chronic muscular tensions.

Rolf (1962) suggests that the human organism as an energy mass is subject to gravitational law. As a plastic medium, capable of change, Rolfing attempts to reorganise and balance the body in relation to gravitational forces. This is done by using pressure and stretch techniques on the fascial tissues in a precise sequence of body areas. The beneficial effects are claimed to be physical, emotional, postural and behavioural.

Rolf states:

Our ignorance of the role and significance of fascia is profound. Therefore even in theory it is easy to overlook the possibility that far-reaching changes may be made not only in structural contour, but also in functional manifestation, through better organisation of the layer of superficial fascia which enwraps the body. Experiments demonstrate that drastic (beneficial) changes may be made in the body, solely by stretching, separating and relaxing superficial fascia in an appropriate manner.

Osteopaths have observed and recorded the extent to which all degenerative change in the body, be it muscular, nervous, circulatory or organic, reflects in superficial fascia. Any degree of degeneration, however minor, changes the bulk of the fascia, modifies its thickness and draws it into ridges in areas overlying deeper tensions and rigidities. Conversely, as this elastic envelope is stretched, manipulative mechanical energy is added to it, and the fascial colloid becomes more 'sol' and less 'gel' (Greenman 1989). The biophysics of this process has been discussed in a classic paper by R. B. Taylor (1958):

As a result of the added energy, as well as of a directional contribution in applying it, the underlying structures, including the muscles which determine the placement of the body parts in space, and also their relations to each other, have come a little closer to the normal ('normal' as used here must be differentiated from 'average') – the patient feels 'so much better'.

Fascial stress responses and therapeutic opportunities

Changes in the fascia can result from passive congestion which results in fibrous infiltration and a more 'sol'-like consistency than is the norm. Under healthy conditions a 'gel'-like ground

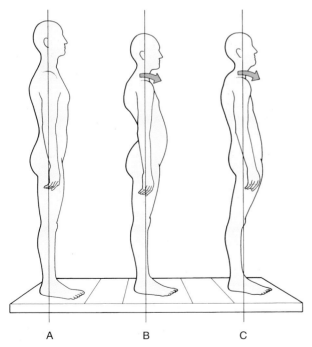

Figure 1.2   Balanced posture (A) compared with two patterns of musculoskeletal imbalance which involve fascial, and general, tissue and joint adaptations.

substance follows the laws of fluid mechanics. Clearly, the more resistive drag there is in a colloidal substance the greater will be the difficulty in normalising this.

Scariati (1991) points out that colloids are not rigid: they conform to the shape of their container, and respond to pressure even though they are not compressible. The amount of resistance they offer increases proportionally to the velocity of motion applied to them, which makes a gentle touch a fundamental requirement if viscous drag and resistance is to be avoided when attempting to produce a release.

When stressful forces (undesirable or therapeutic) are applied to fascia, there is a first reaction in which a degree of slack is allowed to be taken up, followed by what is colloquially referred to as 'creep' – a variable degree of resistance (depending upon the state of the tissues). Creep is an honest term which accurately describes the slow, delayed yet continuous, stretch which occurs in response to a continuously applied load, as long as this is gentle enough to not provoke the resistance of colloidal 'drag'.

Since the fascia comprises a single structure, the implications for body-wide repercussions of distortions in that structure are clear (Fig. 1.2). An example of one possible negative influence of this sort is to be found in the fascial divisions within the cranium, the tentorium cerebelli and falx cerebri which are commonly warped during birthing difficulties (too long or too short a time in the birth canal, forceps delivery etc.) and which are noted in craniosacral therapy as affecting total body mechanics via their influence on fascia (and therefore the musculature) throughout the body (Brookes 1984).

Cantu (1992) describes what he sees as the 'unique' feature of connective tissue as its 'deformation characteristics'. This refers to a combined viscous (permanent) deformation characteristic as well as an elastic (temporary) deformation characteristic. This leads to the clinically important manner in which connective tissue responds to applied mechanical force by first changing in length, followed by some of this change being lost while some remains. The implications of this phenomenon can be seen in the application of stretching techniques to such tissues, as well as in the way they respond to postural and other repetitive insults.

Such changes are not, however, permanent, since collagen (the raw material of fascia/connective tissue) has a limited (300 to 500 day) half-life and just as bone adapts to stresses imposed upon it so will fascia. If therefore negative stresses (posture, use etc.) are modified for the better and/or positive 'stresses' are imposed (manipulation and/or exercise for example) dysfunctional connective tissue can usually be improved over time (Neuberger 1953).

Cantu and Grodin, in their evaluation of the myofascial complex, conclude that therapeutic approaches which sequence their treatment protocols to involve the superficial tissues (involving autonomic responses) as well as deeper tissues (influencing the mechanical components of the musculoskeletal system) and which also address the factor of mobility (movement), are in tune with the requirements of the body when dysfunctional. NMT, as it will be presented, does take this comprehensive approach, and much that it offers seems to be similar to the myofascial release methods currently receiving so much attention in the USA.

Cathie (1974) maintains that the contractile phase of fascial activity supersedes all of its other qualities. The attachments of fascia, he states, have a tendency to shorten after periods of marked activity which are followed by periods of inactivity and the ligaments become tighter and thicker with advancing age. The properties of fascia (connective tissue) that he regards as being important to therapeutic consideration are listed as follows:

1. It is richly endowed with nerve endings.
2. It has the ability to contract and to stretch elastically.
3. It gives extensive muscular attachment.
4. It supports and stabilises, thus enhancing the postural balance of the body.
5. It is vitally involved in all aspects of motion.
6. It aids in circulatory economy, especially of venous and lymphatic fluids.

7. Fascial change will precede many chronic degenerative diseases.
8. Fascial changes predispose towards chronic tissue congestion.
9. Such chronic passive congestion precedes the formation of fibrous tissue, which then proceeds to an increase in hydrogen ion concentration of articular and periarticular structures.
10. Fascial specialisations produce definite stress bands.
11. Sudden stress (trauma) on fascial tissue will often result in a burning type of pain.
12. Fascia is a major arena of inflammatory processes.
13. Fluids and infectious processes often travel along fascial planes.
14. The CNS is surrounded by fascial tissue (dura mater) which, in the skull, attaches to bone, so that dysfunction in these tissues can have profound and widespread effects.

Greenman (1989) describes how fascia responds to loads and stress in both a plastic and an elastic manner, its response depending upon the type, duration and amount of the load. The responses to either acute injury or repetitive microtrauma (short leg imbalance, for example) are, according to Greenman, likely to follow a sequence of inflammation which subsequently leads to absorption of inflammatory fluids into the superficial fascia, as well as into tight compartmentalised areas in the deep fascia – with this latter event being both palpable and detrimental.

Another variable (apart from the nature of the stress load) which influences the way fascia responds to stress, and what the individual feels of the process, relates to the number of collagen and elastic fibres contained in any given region. Neural receptors within the fascia report to the central nervous system as part of any adaptation process – with the Pacinian corpuscles being particularly important in terms of their involvement in reflex responses.

Other neural input into the pool of activity, and responses to biomechanical stress, involve specialised fascial structures such as tendons and ligaments which contain highly specialised and sensitive mechanoreceptors and proprioceptive reporting stations.

Changes which occur in connective tissue, and which result in such alterations as thickening, shortening, calcification and erosion, may be a painful result of sudden or sustained tension or traction. Cathie (1974) points out that many trigger points (he calls them trigger 'spots') correspond to points where nerves pierce fascial investments. The causes of derangement may therefore be seen to result from faulty muscular activity, alteration in bony relationships, visceral positional change (e.g. visceroptosis) and the adoption of unnatural positions. All these can be sustained, repetitive causes or single, violently induced changes. Chemical (nutritional) factors influencing fascial behaviour should also be considered for, as Pauling (1976) points out, 'Many of the results of deprivation of ascorbic acid involve a deficiency in connective tissue which is largely responsible for the strength of bones, teeth, skin, of the body and which consists of the fibrous protein collagen'.

He goes on to point out that, in deficiency of vitamin C, this binding material becomes less efficient and more fluid. Pauling concludes that the effectiveness of vitamin C in helping the body contain viral particles may to some extent be a result of its strengthening action on connective tissue, which would impede the motion of viral particles through tissue. This illustrates again the ubiquitous nature of the musculoskeletal tissues in general and fascia in particular, and the profound effect on the body economy of dysfunction in any of its myriad components.

Modern techniques of electron and phase microscopy have been used to study myofascial biochemistry activity showing that much of the fascia and connective tissue is built of tubular structures. Erlinghauser (1959) has shown that lymph and cerebrospinal fluid spreads throughout the body via these channels. The implications of this knowledge have not yet been fully realised or investigated by physiologists but play a large part in the theories (and practice) of cranial and craniosacral therapists (Upledger 1988).

Having briefly scanned the influences of stress, both short and long term, on the musculoskeletal system, and of the varying ways in which the soft tissues respond – acutely, chronically and with variations based on their structure – and before looking more closely at reflex phenomena, notably myofascial trigger points which result from such stress, a brief introduction to neuromuscular technique will provide an indication of its potential for dealing with such soft tissue distress.

REFERENCES

Alexander F M 1957 The use of the self. Educational Publications
Baldry P 1993 Acupuncture, trigger points and musculoskeletal pain. Churchill Livingstone, Edinburgh
Barlow W 1959 Anxiety and muscle tension pain. British Journal of Clinical Practice 3(5): 339–350
Basmajian J 1974 Muscles alive. Williams and Wilkins, Baltimore
Boadella D 1978 The language of the body in bioenergetic therapy. Journal of the Research Society for Natural Therapeutics
Brookes D 1984 Cranial osteopathy. Thorsons, London
Butler D 1991 Mobilisation of the nervous system. Churchill Livingstone, Melbourne
Buzzell K 1970 The physiological basis of osteopathic medicine. Postgraduate Institute of Osteopathic Medicine and Surgery, New York
Cantu R, Grodin A 1992 Myofascial manipulation. Aspen Publications, Maryland
Cathie A 1974 Selected writings. Academy of Applied Osteopathy Yearbook 1974. Colorado Springs
Chaitow L 1989 Soft tissue manipulation. Thorsons, London
Cyriax J 1962 Textbook of orthopaedic medicine. Cassell
Dicke E 1978 A manual of reflexive therapy. Sydney Simons, Scarsdale, New York
DiGiovanna E 1991 An osteopathic approach to diagnosis and treatment. Lippincott, London
Dvorak J, Dvorak V 1984 Manual medicine – diagnostics. Georg Thiem Verlag, Stuttgart
Eeman L 1947 Cooperative healing. Frederick Muller, London
Engel A et al 1986 Skeletal muscle types in Myology. McGraw-Hill, New York
Erlinghauser R F 1959 Circulation of C.S.F. through connective tissues. Academy of Applied Osteopathy Yearbook, Carmel, California
Feldenkrais M 1977 Awareness through movement. Harper & Row, New York

Frankel V 1980 Basic biomechanics of the skeletal system. Lea and Febiger, Philadelphia

Gray H 1977 Gray's Anatomy, 35th edn. Churchill Livingstone, Edinburgh

Greenman P 1989 Principals of manual medicine. Williams and Wilkins, Baltimore

Grieve G 1985 Mobilisation of the spine. Churchill Livingstone, Edinburgh

Janda V 1982 Introduction to functional pathology of the motor system. Proceedings VII Commonwealth and International Conference on Sport. Physiotherapy in Sport 3: 39

Janda V 1983 Muscle function testing. Butterworths, London

Janda V 1988 In: Grant R (ed.) Physical therapy of the cervical and thoracic spine. Churchill Livingstone, Edinburgh

Jokl P 1984 Muscle and low back pain. Journal of the American Osteopathic Association 84(1): 64–65

Jones L 1980 Strain and counterstrain. Academy of Applied Osteopathy, Colorado Springs

Korr I 1970 The physiological basis of osteopathic medicine. Postgraduate Institute of Osteopathic Medicine, New York

Korr I 1976 Spinal cord as organiser of disease process. Academy of Applied Osteopathy Yearbook, Colorado Springs

Korr I 1978 Neurologic mechanisms in manipulative therapy. Plenum Press, New York

Korr I 1981 Axonal transport and neurotrophic functions in spinal cord as organiser of disease processes (part 4). Academy of Applied Osteopathy (March): 451–458

Latey P 1983 Muscular manifesto. Self-published, London

Lewis Sir T 1942 Pain. New York

Lewit K 1985 Manipulation in rehabilitation of the locomotor system. Butterworths, London

Lewit K 1992 Manipulation in rehabilitation of the locomotor system. Butterworths

Lewit K 1993 Manipulation in rehabilitation of the locomotor system. Butterworths

Lin J-P 1994 Physiological maturation of muscles in childhood. The Lancet 4 June: 1386–1389

Little K E 1969 Toward more effective manipulative management of chronic myofascial strain and stress syndromes. Journal of the American Osteopathic Association 68

McConnell C 1962 Osteopathic Institute of Applied Technique Yearbook 1962, London

Melzack R 1983 The challenge of pain. Penguin, London

Neuberger A et al 1953 Metabolism of collagen. Biochemical Journal 53: 47–52

Pauling L 1976 The common cold and 'flu. W H Freeman

Reich W 1949 Character analysis. Vision Press

Rolf Ida 1962 Structural dynamics. British Academy of Applied Osteopathy Yearbook 1962

Rowlerson A 1981 A novel myosin. Journal of Muscle Research and Cell Motility 2: 415–438

Scariati P 1991 In: DiGiovanna E An osteopathic approach to diagnosis and treatment. Lippincott, London

Selye H 1976 The stress of life. McGraw Hill

Simons D 1987 Myofascial pain due to trigger points. International Rehabilitation Medicine Association Monograph (Series 1), Rademaker OH

Stiles E 1984 Patient Care 15 May: 16–97 and 15 August: 117–164

Stoddard A 1969 Manual of osteopathic practice. Hutchinson, London

Taylor R B 1958 Bioenergetics of man. Academy of Applied Osteopathic Yearbook 1958, Carmel, California

Travell J, Simons D 1983 Myofascial pain and dysfunction (vol 1). Williams and Wilkins, Philadelphia

Travell J, Simons D 1992 Myofascial pain and dysfunction (vol 2). Williams and Wilkins, Philadelphia

Travell J, Simons G 1983/92 Myofascial pain and dysfunction – the trigger point manual. Williams and Wilkins, Baltimore

Upledger J 1988 Craniosacral therapy. Eastland Press, Seattle

Wall P, Melzack R 1989 Textbook of pain. Churchill Livingstone, Edinburgh

Warwick R, Williams P 1973 Gray's anatomy, 3rd edn. W B Saunders

Woo SL-Y et al 1987 Injury and repair of musculoskeletal soft tissues. American Academy of Orthopedic Surgeons Symposium, Savannah GA

2

Introduction to NMT

Origins of NMT

Imagine a palpation technique which becomes a means of therapeutic intervention by virtue of the addition of increased pressure.

Imagine also a palpation technique, which in a non-invasive manner, meets and matches the tone of the tissues it is addressing and sequentially seeks out changes from the norm in almost all accessible (to finger or thumb) areas of the soft tissues.

Imagine this approach as systematically providing information as to tissue-tone, fibrosity, oedema, discrete localised soft tissue changes, areas of altered structure, adhesions or pain – and being able to switch from a painless and pleasant assessment mode to a treatment focus which starts the process of normalising the changes it uncovers.

This is neuromuscular technique (NMT).

The developer of European NMT was Stanley Lief, who was born in Lutzen in the Baltic state of Latvia in the early 1890s. He was one of the five children of Isaac and Riva Lief (Riva was the author's grandfather's eldest sister). The family emigrated to South Africa in the early 1900s where Stanley was given a basic primary school education before starting work in his father's trading store in Roodeport, Transvaal.

Lief's poor health led to an interest in physical culture, one source of which was found in popular health magazines published in the USA. Eventually Lief worked his passage to the USA in order to train under the legendary 'physical culturist' Bernard Macfadden. He qualified in chiropractic and naturopathy before World War I, and was in Britain at its outbreak. After serving in the army he returned to England and worked in institutional 'Nature Cure' (naturopathic) resorts until 1925 when he established his own clinic, Champneys, at Tring in Hertfordshire.

At this world-famous healing resort he established his reputation as a daring and pioneering healer. By using the dietetic, fasting, hydro-therapeutic and physical methods by which naturopathy aims to restore normality to the sick body, he developed a huge following, and it was during his most successful years before World War II that he evolved the technique which this book attempts to describe.

Stanley Lief and his cousin Boris Chaitow, who worked as his assistant at Champneys before and during World War II, developed and refined the uses of NMT. Boris Chaitow was also born in Latvia but grew up in South Africa. He had qualified as an attorney and was in practice with my father when he became inspired by Stanley Lief's example and, with his help, trained as a chiropractor at National College, Chicago before joining the staff at Champneys in 1937. In this book, the basic NMT application, together with a variety of specialised associated soft tissue manipulation techniques, will be presented, as will various reflex systems which fall within the scope of soft tissue treatment in general and NMT in particular. Detailed reference to, and illustrations of, the neurolymphatic reflexes of Chapman, together with illustrations of other reflex patterns such as myofascial trigger points, have therefore been included. NMT, as a modality, may be incorporated into any system of physical medicine. It may (and indeed often should) be used as a treatment on its own, or it may accompany (preceding for preference) manipulative and other physical modalities. Its main use up to the present has been in the hands (literally) of the osteopathic profession; however, many physiotherapists, chiropractors, massage therapists and doctors of physical medicine who have studied and used NMT have found it complementary to their own methods of practice.

Since it offers a simultaneous diagnostic and therapeutic capability, NMT is time-saving, energy-saving and, above all, efficient.

Other soft tissue manipulative methods such as muscle energy technique (MET) and functional positional release approaches (strain/counterstrain for example) are commonly used as part of NMT treatment. The key to the successful use of NMT is an ability to sense accurately what it is that the hands are feeling while at the same time having a clear picture of what the particular movement or technique being employed is aimed at achieving. If the practitioner can learn to 'see' with his hands, and by using them let the patient's body 'tell its own tale', then the intelligent application of the methods described has much to offer towards the recovery of health.

Holistic methods of healing demand that, in order to create the situation for the maintenance or the restoration of health, the individual must be seen as a totality.

It is necessary, therefore, to attempt to recognise the various factors affecting both the internal and external environment of the individual, since these are part of the complex interacting totality which can influence the individual for good or ill. In the end, the body is self-healing, self-repairing and self-maintaining, if the prerequisites for health are present. Emotional stability, nutritional balance, hygiene considerations all play their part, as does structural and mechanical integrity.

A brief history

Neuromuscular technique has evolved over the past 60 years from the original work of Stanley Lief. In the mid-1930s he was seeking for improved means to prepare soft tissue structures for subsequent manipulation. He had studied the work of Rabagliatti whose book *Initis* influenced Lief's interest in connective tissue problems. He also became aware of (and studied) the work of a Dr Dewanchand Varma, a practitioner of Ayurvedic manipulation (Varma called his method 'Pranotherapy') who was practising in Paris. In Varma's book *The Human Machine and Its Forces* (Varma 1938) he states:

We have discovered that the circulation of the nervous currents, slows down occasionally because of the obstruction caused by adhesions; the muscular fibres harden and the nervous currents can no longer pass through them. We have demonstrated effective and positive methods designed to restore nervous equilibrium which promotes the healthy circulation of blood, so that new tissues begin to be built up again. Our method of treatment, by the removal of all obstacles to the flow of nervous current, allows energy to proceed unimpeded.

Lief found various of Varma's techniques useful and out of these ideas and methods developed his own soft tissue approach – NMT. Lief's cousin Boris Chaitow describes this early development of NMT as follows (Chaitow, personal communication, 1983):

In the middle of the 1930s Stanley Lief realised that the integrity of a joint was to a great extent related to the character of the tissues surrounding the joint, related to muscle, tendons, ligaments, blood and nerve supply etc. He felt that in order the better to achieve effective mobility and integrity of function of joints – particularly in the spine but also in all bony articular relationships – it was advisable to normalise, as best one could, the adjacent soft tissues by removing any function-interfering factors, such as tensions, contractions, adhesions, spasms, fibrositic contractures etc., with appropriate application of fingers and hands to those tissues. To this end the neuromuscular technique was evolved to cover every possible type of lesion in whatever part of the body (articular, soft tissue, abdominal, glandular, nervous, vascular etc).

It so happened that at that particular time Stanley Lief had heard of a well-known Indian practitioner named Varma operating in Paris, who was applying an unusual but very effective soft-tissue technique on patients with remarkable benefits. Lief decided to arrange to have a series of treatments on himself from Varma, and finally persuaded the latter to teach him this specialised technique. Much as he appreciated the method used by Varma, he felt it could be improved, and began to develop and subsequently practised the method for which he devised the name of 'Neuro-muscular Technique'. This name was an accurate definition of the purpose of the method he evolved from the cruder technique used by Varma. NMT involved an application of hands and fingers to the appropriate areas of soft tissue related to the affected bony articulations, as well as all other areas of soft tissue which his sensitive fingers found to be abnormal in texture. This enables adverse factors in such tissue to be corrected to allow the full function of muscles and nerves to be re-established. In doing so the double benefits are achieved in improving nerve and blood circulation, improving texture of muscle tissue and in being better able to get effective results in manipulating the bony articulations involved, and assuring lasting integrity of their normal function.

Stanley Lief also maintained that joint lesions were not the only factors in the interference in nerve force integrity, but that tensions, contractions, adhesions, muscle spasms and fibrositic contractures in soft tissues could in themselves constitute primary factors in disease (symptom) causation by reducing effective nerve and blood circulation. To this end he developed his diagnostic sensitivity with his fingers so that in a few seconds of palpation over any area of the body, he was able to assess abnormalities present in relation to tensions, adhesions and spasms.

The body's integrity, and its functional efficiency, depends not only on its chemistry influenced by the nature of the food and drink we consume, but also on the effective nerve and blood circulation free of mechanical and functional obstructions. To this second vital purpose there is no formula devised by the osteopathic or chiropractic professions that will more effectively achieve the optimum result than the philosophy and technique devised by Stanley Lief. There is no single part of the body that he was not able to apply his method to to achieve remarkable physiological responses.

Stanley Lief's son, Peter (also a naturopath, chiropractor and osteopath) has described (Lief 1963) the 'neuro-muscular' lesion as being associated with:

1. Congestion of the local connective tissues
2. Disturbance of the acid-base balance of the connective tissues
3. Fibrous infiltration (adhesions)
4. Chronic muscular contractions or hyper- or hypotrophic (tone) changes.

Aetiology of the neuromuscular lesion, according to Stanley and Peter Lief, includes a number of causative factors, giving rise to neuromuscular lesions, which may include:

1. Fatigue, exhaustion, bad posture
2. Local trauma
3. Systemic toxaemia (lack of exercise and oxygen)
4. Dietetic deficiencies
5. Psychosomatic causes bringing about muscular tensions.

The presence of a 'lesion' (current terminology would define this as an area of somatic dysfunction) is always revealed by an area of hypersensitivity to pressure. It is remarkable to note just how close to the defining of causes and characteristics of myofascial trigger points Lief came, although operating many years before the research of Travell and Simons (see Ch. 3).

TISSUES INVOLVED IN NMT

Boris Chaitow and Peter Lief have both taken part in the development and evolution of the theory and application of NMT as first described by Stanley Lief. Another distinguished British naturopath/osteopath who worked with them, Brian Youngs, has given the following descriptive overview of the tissues involved in NMT (Youngs 1962):

Site of application

As the technique (NMT) operates primarily on connective tissue it will usually be concentrated at those areas where such tissue is most dense, e.g. muscular origins and insertions, especially the broad aponeurotic insertions. The most frequent sites are the superior curved line of the occiput, the numerous insertions and origins of the large, medium and small muscles which attach to the vertebral column; the iliac-crest insertions; the intercostal insertions and abdominal-muscle insertions. Nevertheless, the technique can of course be applied to any area which requires it – head, face, wrists, etc. Connective tissue is, after all, ubiquitous.

To understand the therapeutic effect of the technique one must have some knowledge of the pathophysiology of the tissue upon which it operates. Connective tissue consists of a matrix containing cells and fibres. It was largely ignored until recently, but has now been made the subject of close study – and even international conferences – in regard to its structure and functions. Dr Rabagliatti, 45 years ago,[1] was so interested and far-seeing that his book, *Initis*, contained concepts the general truth of which is being proved today. He was, however, a lone voice and because he held unorthodox ideas he was, typically, ignored.

The ubiquity of connective tissue caused Dr Rabagliatti to analogise it to the ether – as the medium for, as he termed it, 'the zoodynamic life force'.

Through the connective tissues' planes run the trunks and plexuses of veins, arteries, nerves, and lymphatics. Connective tissue is the support for the structural and, therefore, functional relationships of these systems.

Chemical structure

Briefly, the matrix consists of a jelly-like ground substance in which the fibres, cells, vessels, etc., lie.

This ground substance is the 'physical expression of the *milieu interieure*' intervening everywhere between the blood and lymph vessels and the metabolising cells; it plays a major role in the transport, storage and exchange of water and electrolytes. The chemical structure is essentially polysaccharide, hyaluronic acid, chondroitin sulphuric acid, chondroitin sulphate and chondroitin itself, together with proteins which contain a considerable amount of the amino acid tyrosine, which forms the majority of the thyroxine molecule.

The fibres are white fibrous (collagen), yellow (elastin), and reticulin. The collagen fibres are also protein and polysaccharide in composition and are stabilised chemically by the presence of the ground substance constituents. The presence of chondroitin sulphate, for example, renders the enzymatic breakdown of collagen much more difficult. The importance of this point will become more clear later. The formation of fibres appears to be due to a precipitation of fibre constituents by serum glycoproteins under the influence of adrenocorticotrophic hormone.

Reticulin contains more polysaccharide than collagen, and some lipid also. Elastin is also protein and polysaccharide in composition. Sulphur is a constituent of all three. Cells include fibroblasts, mast cells, macrophages and others.

A function of circulation

The nature and composition of connective tissue is a function of circulation. Circulatory efficiency in any area will determine (1) the influx of materials to the area, and (2) the drainage of the area.

Incoming blood leads to the production of lymph and this fluid permeates the ground substance, bringing all the constituents of the blood except the proteins to the connective tissue. Some of these constituents are hormones. Thyroxine, adrenoglucocorticoids and adrenomineralocorticoids are only three of these. Oestrogen and androgens are two more. All these have known effects upon the structure of connective tissue. Thus, a diminution of thyroxine leads to an increase of water retention in most cells and an increase in the quantity of ground substance. The sex hormones also do this, but of most interest to us here are the opposing groups of the adrenocortical hormones. Selye divides these into anti- and pro-inflammatory hormones (A-Cs and P-Cs). These are produced in response to stress situations and they exert both a general and a local effect. By regulating the balance between these two the body can control the ability of the tissues to produce an inflammatory response. But when the A-Cs and the P-Cs are both present in the blood the A-Cs always win the contest, i.e., there is an anti-inflammatory response.

---

[1]Young was writing in the mid-60s.

Stressor stimulus

The A-Cs are produced in response to a stimulus – the stressor. The stressor in neuromuscular technique is pain. Effective technique appears to be accompanied by pain in all (I generalise here deliberately) such conditions (and also in the condition without treatment). Pain is probably due to two factors. A much reduced threshold in the area due to circulatory inhibition enabling a build up to just below the threshold level of Lewis pain substance or, alternatively, a disturbance of electrolyte level (e.g., increase of hydrogen ions or disturbance in the calcium/sodium/potassium balance due to the same circumstances). Consequently pain will be produced by even slight stimulus, let alone the heavier movements of neuromuscular technique. Also, pressure and tension proprioceptors may be overstimulated and pain can result from an over application of any ordinary stimulus.

The A-Cs liberated will produce both general effects (general adaptation syndrome) and local effects (local adaptation syndrome) and their effect is anti-inflammatory, both generally and locally, at the area of application of the stressor, i.e., at the areas of technique application. Consequently, there is a breakdown of collagen fibres and a general decrease in water retention in the ground substance; the congested area is decongested.

What Youngs has described tallies closely with what is now known about the biochemical status of tissues under stress, and particularly of the trigger point entity which will be evaluated in following chapters.

Stanley Lief, albeit inadvertently, provided for the generation of practitioners who were to follow him a tool with which to deal with this pain-producing end-result of the multiple stresses faced by the modern musculoskeletal system.

In the latter part of the life of Stanley Lief, and during the later active years in practice of Boris Chaitow (alive and well and in his late-80s at the time of writing) awareness grew as to other applications of use for NMT, most notably in its potential to identify and commence elimination of myofascial trigger points.

The principal author has over the past 30 years, since working as assistant to Boris Chaitow in the early 1960s, helped to promote knowledge of NMT – particularly in its diagnostic mode – so that it stands today as a major therapeutic instrument for use by manipulative and massage therapists world-wide. The use of NMT as a broadly applicable sequential assessment and treatment tool was enhanced by exposure to the work of Raymond Nimmo in the late 1960s. Nimmo and his 'receptor-tonus' work seems to be a common link between 'European' NMT and American NMT – as described by Judith Walker in this and other segments of the text devoted to the transatlantic perspective of NMT. Detailed descriptions, with additional insights from Boris Chaitow of the means of application of NMT, in both its assessment and treatment modes, will be found in later chapters.

Judith Walker's overview of NMT in the USA

What has today become neuromuscular therapy in the USA was spawned in the late 1970s from receptor-tonus method (the work of the late Dr Raymond Nimmo). Nimmo, a 1926 graduate of Palmer College of Chiropractic, states in his writings that he questioned many of the philosophical and theoretical teachings of his profession (Nimmo 1959). He studied many aspects of classic chiropractic even though he was convinced that adjustment of the spine was not enough to ensure the health of the individual. He also sought out information as to the role which soft tissues play in pain and dysfunction in an attempt to explain the syndromes he was confronted with in his work.

As Nimmo developed his palpation of the muscles, he noted particular points within the muscles which, when pressed, referred pain to various areas. He called these 'noxious generative points' (NGPs). In 1952 Nimmo purchased *Connective Tissue: Transactions of the Second Conference*, (Travell 1952) in which Janet Travell discussed her theories of trigger points. Nimmo found illustrations of referred pain patterns in Travell's work which coincided precisely with his own discoveries. He began working obsessively to develop a sensible treatment plan and states that, as time went by, he learned from others but probably 80 to 90% of the techniques he taught were his own work.

Nimmo's constant striving to prove the physiological basis of his work, complete with integration of neurological laws which gave validity and substance to his principles of practice, derived not only from being in the forefront of a newly-emerging profession, but also from the fact that his interest in the soft tissue component of the body placed him at the very fringes of the teachings of that profession.

He faced peers at a time when they were attempting to validate the principles of chiropractic and asked them to question the very basis of their beliefs. His work endured and many health care practitioners who studied with him carried the work forward, under a variety of names.

In 1979 Paul St John, who had studied receptor-tonus methodology with Nimmo, published material relating to similar techniques which he called neuromuscular therapy (NMT). His concepts were influenced by not only Nimmo (Vannerson 1971), but also Travell and Simons (1983), Mariano Racabado, Leon Chaitow, Rene Cailliet (1977), Aaron Mattes, John Barnes, John Upledger and others through their writings and seminars. Judith Walker's professional association with St John in 1984 led to revisions of previous concepts, with significant changes in treatment techniques and teaching materials, which came to include the influence of posture and craniosacral methods. During this phase, the work of Janet Travell and David Simons had enormous influence. Their book *Myofascial pain – A trigger point manual*, (Travell & Simons 1983) and numerous articles by them, began to explain in greater detail the background to what Nimmo had taught. In 1989 St John and Walker separated their work and both continue to teach neuromuscular therapy. The approaches which they have taken, although still containing elements of Nimmo's original work, have now diverged, with St John's work focusing on structural homeostasis of the body and cranium by applying the law of cause and effect and Walker's incorporating a systematic approach towards pain relief which addresses six physiological factors: ischaemia, trigger points, nerve compression/entrapment, postural distortion (biomechanics), nutrition and emotional wellbeing (stress reduction). Judith Walker has provided a detailed overview of American NMT in its current stage of evolution in Chapter 11.

REFERENCES

Cailliet R 1977 soft tissue pain and disability. F A Davis, Philadelphia
Lief P 1963 British Naturopathic Journal 5(10)
Nimmo R (undated) The receptor and tonus control method. The Receptor 1(2)
Nimmo R 1959 Factor X. The Receptor (1)4
Travell J 1952 Connective tissue: transactions of the second conference. The Josiah Macy Jr Foundation, New York

Travell J, Simons D 1983 Myofascial pain and dysfunction: the trigger point manual. Williams & Wilkins, Baltimore
Vannerson J, Nimmo R 1971 Specificity and the law of facilitation in the nervous system. The Receptor 2(1)
Varma D 1935 The human machine and its forces. Health For All, London
Youngs B 1962 Physiological background of neuro-muscular technique. British Naturopathic Journal 5(6): 176–190

3

Myofascial and other reflex phenomena

PAIN PATTERNS

Myofascial trigger points are a major cause of sustained pain and dysfunction according to Melzack and Wall, leading researchers into pain, and indeed are stated by them to be a part of all chronic pain conditions (Wall & Melzack 1989).

The multitude of descriptions and classifications of reflex pain patterns – many of which are outlined in the following chapters – demand a brief review of the possible mechanisms.

The first need is to differentiate between pain and referred symptoms which are of a spinal, nerve root, origin and those which have different sources.

Difference between referred phenomena and radicular pain

Pain and other root syndrome effects deriving from damaged or dysfunctional vertebral or intervertebral structures need to be differentiated from the non-radicular pain and symptoms which derive from reflexogenic activity – myofascial trigger points, for example.

The key characteristics of radicular dysfunction from, for example, a herniated disc, will include (Dubs 1950, Dvorak & Dvorak 1984):

- Pain located in the regions supplied by the nerve roots from the segment(s) involved
- A loss of sensitivity in the appropriate dermatomes related to the segment(s) involved
- A loss of motor power – possibly to the point of paralysis – of the muscle innervated by the nerve roots involved and possible atrophy

- Disturbances of the deep tendon reflexes in the related areas.

The diagnosis of the presence of such dysfunction requires expert neurological assessment; however, practitioners and therapists should be aware of these key signs, which alert them to the possibility that nerve root syndromes may be a feature of the patient's problem.

Non-radicular patterns of referred pain

Dvorak has described five variations on the theme of referred symptomatology, different ways of seeing the same phenomena, aside from nerve root syndromes (Dvorak & Dvorak 1984).

These are:

1. Referred pain – which includes the findings described by researchers such as Lewis (1938), Kellgren (1938), Hockaday and Whittey (1967) which demonstrated that mechanical and chemical stimulation to various spinal structures produces referred pain. This is discussed further in this chapter (p. 30).

2. Myofascial trigger points, which are discussed extensively in this chapter, and which form the major focus of neuromuscular technique application in North America.

3. Pseudoradicular syndromes which Brugger (1962) describes as being quite distinct from root syndromes and which derive from a 'nociceptive somatomotoric blocking effect' occurring in tissues such as joint capsules, tendon origins and other local (to joint) tissues. These painful reflex effects are noted in muscles and their tendinous junctions as well as the skin – which Brugger calls 'tendomyosis' – defined as, 'the reflexogenic functional change in the muscle in the presence of concurrent functionally dependent muscle pain'. Dvorak includes in this category of referred pain and symptoms the phenomena of viscerosomatic and somatovisceral influences, in which, for example, organ dysfunction is said to produce tendomyotic changes (Korr 1975). Some aspects of these phenomena form part of the discussion of facilitation in this chapter (p. 30).

4. Tender points, as described by Lawrence Jones, which Dvorak equates with the tender points described by Kellgren (see Ch. 4, p. 58, for more on Jones work) are seen to be spontaneously arising areas of tenderness related to acute or chronic strains, usually located in those soft tissues shortened at the time of the strain.

5. Spondylogenic reflexes, knowledge of which Dvorak describes as being based on empirical clinical observation which demonstrates relationships between the axial skeleton and the peripheral soft tissues which 'are not easily explained on the basis of radicular, vascular or humoral reasoning'. The effects of these reflexes includes 'demonstrable zones of irritation ... which are painful swellings, tender upon pressure, located in the musculofascial tissue in topographically well-defined sites' (Sutter 1975).

Dvorak acknowledges what is increasingly obvious – that these different classifications and descriptions are focusing on the self-same phenomena, with terminology and interpretations being the variables, rather than there being a host of different physiological patterns of response to stress and trauma.

In this context earlier research into referred pain is worth re-evaluating, since it highlights basic facts of which many have lost sight.

Speransky

Speransky, in his classic book *A Basis for the Theory of Medicine* (Speransky 1943) demonstrated clearly that: 'From any nerve point it is easy to bring into action nerve mechanisms, the functioning of which terminates at the periphery, in changes of a bio-physico-chemical character.' And further: 'Justification exists for the thesis that any nerve point, not excluding peripheral nerve structures, can become the originator of neurodystrophic processes, serving as the temporary nerve centre of these processes.'

Speransky went on: 'It is obvious from this [evidence] that the irritation of any point of the complex network of the nervous system, can evoke changes, not only in the adjacent parts, but also in remote regions of the organism.'

Kellgren

Following on from the pioneering work of Sir Thomas Lewis, the researcher J. H. Kellgren performed a series of studies in the late 1930s which deserve our attention (Kellgren 1938, Kellgren 1939, Lewis 1938).

Kellgren effectively showed that by irritating fascia and muscle (using himself and volunteers) he could produce referred sensations in other structures. For example, among his early findings was evidence that a saline injection into the occipital muscles would produce a headache while similar irritation to the masseter muscle produced a toothache.

Kellgren concluded that such distribution of pain usually followed segmental pathways, although he modified this position when he applied his studies to clinical work, at which time he not only identified localised, exquisitely painful spots which referred painful symptoms to distant areas, but also noted that the distribution of pain from such spots did not in fact always follow peripheral neural pathways. He also showed that a local anaesthetic injection into such spots could obliterate the referred pain sensations.

Kellgren (1939) stated:

Superficial fascia (of the back) and supraspinous ligaments induce local pain when stimulated, while stimulation of the superficial portions of the interspinous ligaments and superficial muscles result in diffuse pain. Deep muscles, ligaments and periostium of the apophyseal joints as well as the joints themselves can cause referred pain according to segmental innervation when stimulated [saline solution or mechanical stimulus].

Other research at that time (1940s) indicated that there was not always a predictable pattern of pain distribution from such experiments (Feinstein 1954) (Fig. 3.1).

Research by many others in the 1940s, continuing up to the present, has further investigated referred patterns of pain which do not seem to follow neurological pathways, or even known patterns of viscerally caused pain – or for that matter the common acupuncture pathways as described in traditional Chinese medicine – myofascial trigger points.

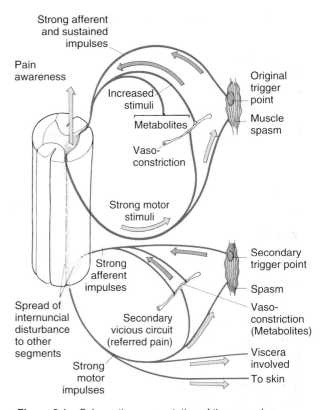

Figure 3.1 Schematic representation of the secondary spread of neurologically induced influences deriving from acute or chronic soft tissue dysfunction, and involving trigger point activity and/or spasm.

Evans

Evans in discussing reflex pain, describes the mechanism as follows:

A prolonged bombardment of pain impulses sets up a vicious circle of reflexes spreading through a pool of many neuron connections upward, downward and even across the spinal cord and perhaps reaching as high as the thalamus itself. Depending upon the extent of the pool (internuncial pool), we detect the phenomena of pain and sympathetic disturbances a long distance from the injured (trigger) area of the body and occasionally even spread to the contralateral side.

Dittrich

Dittrich (1954) has shown a constant pattern of fibrosis of subfascial tissue, with adhesions between this and the overlying muscle fascia, in a number of distinctive and common pain patterns. For example in what he calls the 'mid-sacral syndrome' which develops from sacral lesions, referred pain is almost always present in the buttock and sometimes in the thigh, leg or foot. Referred tenderness is elicited in the lower part of the buttock. The fibrous adhesions (trigger area) are found at the level of the 3rd sacral vertebra near the spine.

In the 'mid-lumbar syndrome' he showed that there is referred pain and tenderness in the lower lumbar, upper sacral and sacroiliac regions. The trigger point is found over the lateral third of the sacrospinalis muscle at the level of the upper margin of the iliac crest.

The 'latissimus-dorsi syndrome' could result from irritation of the aponeurosis of this muscle at either of the sites of injury, sacral or lumbar, mentioned above. Referred pain would develop in the sclerotonic distributions of the 6th, 7th, and 8th cervical nerves.

Dittrich pointed out that pathological changes at the two sites have been discovered by operative findings. His technique was to surgically remove these triggers or to obliterate the triggers by injection of local anaesthetic. No concern is expressed as to the mechanical, postural or other reasons that may have produced them, nor any mention made of more conservative manipulative methods of normalisation.

The presence of 'fibrosed subfascial tissue' supports the theories of Stanley Lief and Boris Chaitow and their use of NMT in treating such problems (see Ch. 2, p. 21). The locale of these, close to bony insertions, further supports the rationale behind neuromuscular technique.

It seems that soft tissue lesions, characterised by fibrosis of subfascial tissue (fat etc.) with fibrous connections between the structure and the overlying fascia, can initiate sensory irritation which produce referred pain and tenderness. In addition, autonomic nervous involvement may be activated to produce vasomotor, trophic, visceral or metabolic changes. Symptoms will disappear when the offending lesion is normalised by whatever method. However, a system that both corrects the offending trigger and attempts

to prevent its recurrence would seem to offer greater clinical benefits. Leaving aside myofascial trigger points for the moment allows for a survey of some of the other reflex patterns which are pertinent to this text.

Gutstein

Gutstein (1956) showed that conditions such as ametropia may result from changes in the neuromuscular component of the craniocervical area, as well as from more distant conditions involving the pelvis or shoulder girdle. He states:

Myopia is the long-term effect of pressure of extra-ocular muscles in the convergence effort of accommodation involving spasm of the ciliary muscles, with resultant elongation of the eyeball. A sequential relationship has been shown between such a condition and muscular spasm of the neck.

Normalisation of these muscles by manipulation relieves eye symptoms as well as fascial, dorsolumbar and abdominal tenderness. Gutstein terms these reflexes 'myodysneuria' and suggests that the reference phenomena of such spots or triggers would include pain, modifications of pain, itching, hypersensitivity to physiological stimuli, spasm, twitching, weakness and trembling of striated muscles; hyper- or hypotonus of smooth muscle of blood vessels, and of internal organs; hyper- or hyposecretion of visceral, sebaceous and sudatory glands. Somatic manifestations may also occur in response to visceral stimuli of corresponding spinal levels (Gutstein 1944).

Many such trigger areas are dormant and asymptomatic. Gutstein's method of treatment is the injection of an anaesthetic solution into the trigger area. He indicates, however, that where accessible (e.g. muscular insertions in the cervical area) the chilling of these areas combined with pressure will yield good results. This is in line with Mennell's work (p. 37) and fits into the field of neuromuscular technique.

Amongst the patterns of vasomotor sebaceous, sudatory and gastrointestinal dysfunction mentioned by Gutstein (1944) are the following, all of which relate to reflex trigger points or 'myodysneuria' (fibrositis/fibromyalgia):

1. Various patterns of vasomotor abnormality such as coldness, pallor, redness, cyanosis etc. These variations in response to stimulation relate to the fact that most organs respond to weak stimuli by an increase in activity and to very strong stimuli by inhibiting activity. Menopausal hot flushes are one example and these seem often to be linked with musculoskeletal pain. Gutstein found that obliteration of overt and silent triggers in the occipital, cervical, interscapular, sternal and epigastric regions was accompanied by years of alleviation of premenopausal, menopausal and late menopausal symptoms. Proponents of NMT have long emphasised the importance of normalising these very structures.

2. Gutstein maintains that normalisation of skin secretion, and therefore of hair and skin texture and appearance, may be altered for the better by the removal of active trigger areas in the cervical and interscapular areas.

3. The conditions of hyper-, hypo- and anhidrosis may accompany vasomotor and sebaceous dysfunction. Gutstein noted that abolition of excessive perspiration as well as anhidrosis followed adequate treatment.

4. Gutstein quotes a number of practitioners who have achieved success in treating gastrointestinal dysfunctions by treating trigger areas. Some of these were treated by procaine injection, others by pressure techniques and massage. The abdominal wall lends itself to this latter procedure as evidenced by the work of Cornelius (1909) whose treatment was not dissimilar to that of Lief's NMT.

Among the conditions which have responded to such treatment are: Pylorospasm, bad breath, heartburn, regurgitation, nausea, abdominal distension, constipation, nervous diarrhoea etc. Gutstein (1944) tried to denote localised functional sensory and/or motor abnormalities of musculoskeletal tissue (comprising muscle, fascia, tendon, bone and joint) as myodysneuria (now known as fibromyalgia – formerly known as 'fibrositis' and 'muscular rheumatism'). He sees the causes of such changes as multiple and among these are:

1. Acute and chronic infections which, it is postulated, stimulate sympathetic nerve activity via their toxins.

2. Excessive heat or cold, changes in atmospheric pressure and draughts.

3. Mechanical injuries, both major and repeated minor microtraumas. Postural strain, unaccustomed exercises etc., which may predispose towards future changes by lowering the threshold for future stimuli (facilitation).

4. Allergic and endocrine factors which can cause imbalance in the autonomic nervous system.

5. Inherited factors making adjustment to environmental factors difficult.

6. Arthritic changes: since muscles are the active components of the musculoskeletal system it is logical to assume that their circulatory state has influence over bones and joints. Spasm in muscle may contribute towards osteoarthritic changes and such changes may produce further neuromuscular changes which themselves produce new symptoms.

7. Visceral diseases may intensify and precipitate somatic symptoms in the distribution of their spinal and adjacent segments.

In these examples of Gutstein's concept we can see strong echoes of the facilitation hypothesis in osteopathic medicine, and it seems likely that they are describing the same set of circumstances leading to hyperreactive responses – and all this leads to in terms of pain and dysfunction.

Diagnosis of myodysneuria was made according to some of the following criteria:

- A varying degree of muscular tension and contraction is usually present although sometimes adjacent, apparently unaffected tissue is more painful.
- Sensitivity to pressure or palpation of affected muscles and their adjuncts.

Marked hypertonicity may require the application of deep pressure to demonstrate tenderness.

Travell and Bigelow

Travell and Bigelow produced evidence that supports much of what Gutstein had reported

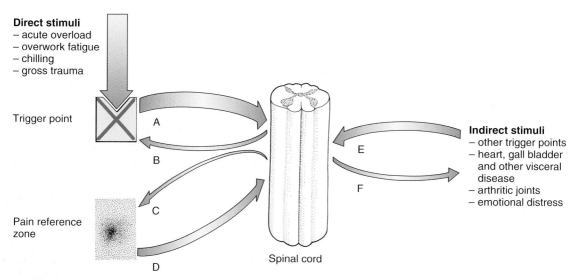

Direct stimuli
– acute overload
– overwork fatigue
– chilling
– gross trauma

Trigger point

A

B

C

Pain reference
zone

D

Spinal cord

Indirect stimuli
– other trigger points
– heart, gall bladder
  and other visceral
  disease
– arthritic joints
– emotional distress

E

F

Figure 3.2   Direct stress influence can affect the hyper reactive neural structure of a myofascial trigger point, leading to increased activity (A–B) as well as referring sensations (pain, paraesthesia, increased sympathetic activity) to a target area (C–D) which feed back into the cord to increase the background stress load. Other stimuli reach the cord from distant trigger points and additional dysfunctional areas (E–F).

(Travell & Bigelow 1947). They indicate that high-intensity stimuli from active trigger areas produce, by reflex, prolonged vasoconstriction with partial ischaemia in localised areas of the brain, spinal cord, or peripheral nerve structures (Fig. 3.2). There might result a wide pattern of dysfunction affecting almost any organ of the body. The phenomenon of hysteria with symptoms as varied as disordered vision, respiration, motor power and cutaneous sensation, were often mediated by afferent neural impulses from trigger areas in skeletal muscle. These triggers, when similarly located, produced the same pattern of clinical effects, whether activated in one patient by psychogenic factors or in another by different factors (e.g. mechanical or traumatic). It is worth recording that Travell has shown that the effect of a trigger point on the muscle housing it is to produce weakness of contraction without atrophy, and that this is often accompanied by a decreased range of movement in associated joints (Travell 1981).

UNDERSTANDING FACILITATION

If we are to make sense of the phenomenon of myofascial trigger points there is a need to grasp

the processes which lead to hyperirritability and hyperreactivity of specific neural structures – facilitation. Trigger points are localised areas of soft tissue dysfunction which negatively influence distant target areas, and which evolve in a similar manner to that observed when spinal segments become facilitated due to stress of one sort or another.

To understand trigger points we need to understand spinal facilitation first.

Facilitation occurs in both spinal and paraspinal tissues (segmental facilitation) as well as in discrete local areas of muscles, mainly near their origins and insertions but also close to their bellies and in areas where fascial stress occurs due to external influences and forces (myofascial trigger points). Understanding facilitation helps us to see how the different classification systems, all describing variations on the same phenomenon of referred pain – listed by Dvorak and described earlier in this chapter (p. 26) – are held together aetiologically.

Professor Michael Patterson (1976) explains segmental (spinal) facilitation as follows:

The concept of the facilitated segment states that because of abnormal afferent or sensory inputs to a particular area of the spinal cord, that area is kept in a state of constant increased excitation. This facilitation allows normally ineffectual or subliminal stimuli to become effective in producing efferent output from the facilitated segment, causing both skeletal and visceral organs innervated by the affected segment to be maintained in a state of overactivity. It is probable that the 'osteopathic lesion', or somatic dysfunction with which a facilitated segment is associated, is the direct result of the abnormal segmental activity as well as being partially responsible for the facilitation.

A facilitated segment therefore emerges from a prolonged period during which abnormal or altered inputs from a single source (or more than one source) of irritation impinging on the spinal cord, keep the interneurons or motorneurons of that spinal segment in a constant state of excitement, thus allowing normally ineffectual inputs to produce outputs to all organs receiving innervation from the excited area. This concept implies that the spinal cord is a relatively passive mediator of the influences imposed on it and that the neural paths act as communicators of that activity (Denslow et al 1949).

Recent research on spinal functions seems to indicate, however, that the spinal cord, besides being the determiner of where abnormal activity is sent by virtue of predetermined pathways, may participate actively in either controlling abnormal or unusually intense inputs, or amplifying and retaining such inputs in certain circumstances (Korr 1986).

Initially, only intensities of afferent input above a certain level would result in increased sensitivity of the spinal pathway. Inputs of lower intensity would either cause no alterations, or would cause an actual decrease in sensitivity as a protective mechanism against undue changes in homeostatic processes. It is apparent that the potential for sensitisation by different types of afferent inputs may differ widely. Thus, inputs from pain receptors may sensitise the pathway at low levels because of the properties of the initial synapses between pain afferent fibres and interneurons. In this event an initially protective increase in response might occur, followed eventually by detrimental facilitation of a segment. On the other hand, inputs from joint receptors seem to have a less dramatic effect at similar input levels (Dowling 1991). It is

now known that emotional arousal would also affect the susceptibility of the pathways to sensitisation (Baldry 1993). The increase in descending influences from the emotionally aroused subject would result in an increase in toxic excitement in the pathways and allow all additional inputs to produce sensitisation at low intensities. Thus, highly emotional people, or those in a highly emotional situation, would be expected to show a higher incidence of facilitation of spinal pathways.

Since the higher brain centres do influence the tonic levels of the spinal paths, it might be expected also that physical training and mental attitudes would tend to alter the tonic excitability as well, reducing the person's susceptibility to sensitisation from everyday stress. Thus the athlete would be expected to withstand a comparatively high level of afferent input prior to experiencing the self-perpetuating results of sensitisation.

A further corollary of the hypothesis is that slowly developing conditions, or slowly increasing inputs, would result in less sensitisation at high levels than sudden inputs. The slow development of a chronic source of increased sensory input initially would cause habituation, resulting in resistance to sensitisation until the input level was abnormally high. On the other hand, sudden increases in input, such as a sudden mechanical stress, would be expected to produce sensitisation of the neural pathways most rapidly.

Korr

The premier researcher into facilitation over the past half century has been Irwin Korr (Korr 1970, Korr 1976). In early studies he demonstrated, for example, that if readings were taken of resistance to electricity in the paraspinal skin of an individual it could be shown that there were often marked differences, with one side showing normal resistance and the other showing reduced resistance (facilitated area).

When 'stress' was applied elsewhere in the body and the two areas of the spine were monitored, it was the area of facilitation, where electrical resistance was reduced, that showed a

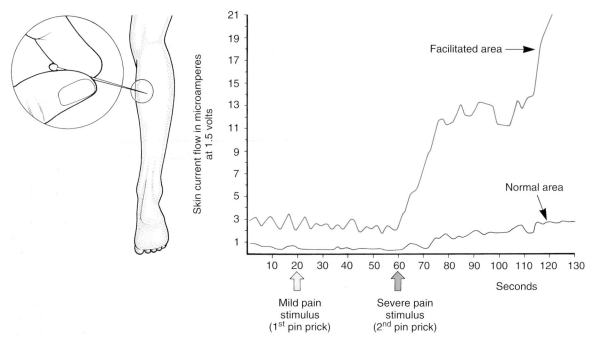

Figure 3.3   Pain stimuli produce a marked reaction in the facilitated area (red line) and little reaction in the normal area (black line).

dramatic rise in electrical (i.e., neurological) activity. In one experiment volunteers had pins inserted into one calf muscle in order to gauge the effect in the paraspinal areas under investigation – with the spinal areas being monitored for electrical activity. While almost no increase occurred in the normal region, the facilitated area showed enormously enhanced neurological activity after 60 seconds (Fig. 3.3) (Korr 1977).

The implications of this and hundreds of similar studies are that any form of stress impacting the individual, be it climatic, chemical, emotional, physical or anything else, would produce just such a rise in neurological output from facilitated areas.

In many instances involving spinal segmental facilitation there is a chronic degree of neurological bombardment resulting from internal organ dysfunction. For example, it is almost always possible to predict that cardiovascular disease is present (or will soon be present) when two or more segments of the spine in the region of T2, 3, 4 display tense, rigid, 'board-like' characteristics on palpation, especially if these tissues do not respond to normal efforts to reduce their hypertonicity (Beal 1983).

Viscerosomatic reflexes

Many of the various systems involving reflexively active points described in this and the next chapter, such as Chapman's reflexes and Bennett's reflexes, as well as trigger points, may involve viscerosomatic reflex activity.

Beal

Myron Beal (1985) has described this phenomenon as resulting from afferent stimuli, arising from dysfunction of a visceral nature. The reflex is initiated by afferent impulses arising from visceral receptors, which are transmitted to the dorsal horn of the spinal cord, where they synapse with interconnecting neurons. The stimuli are then conveyed to sympathetic and motor efferents, resulting in changes in the somatic tissues, such as skeletal muscle, skin and blood vessels.

Abnormal stimulation of the visceral efferent neurons may result in hyperasthesia of the skin, and associated vasomotor, pilomotor and sudomotor changes. Similar stimuli of the ventral horn cells may result in reflex rigidity of the somatic musculature. Pain may result from such changes.

The degree of stimulus required, in any given case, to produce such changes will differ, since factors such as prior facilitation of the particular segment, as well as the response of higher centres, will differ from person to person.

In many cases it is suggested, by Korr and others, that viscerosomatic reflex activity may be noted before any symptoms of visceral change are evident, and that this phenomenon is therefore of potential diagnostic and prognostic value. *1st signs of Viscerosmatic Reflex*

The first signs of viscerosomatic reflexive influences are vasomotor reactions (increased skin temperature), sudomotor (increased moisture of the skin), skin textural changes (e.g. thickening), increased subcutaneous fluid, and increased contraction of muscle. The value of light skin palpation in identifying areas of facilitation cannot be too strongly emphasised (Lewit 1992).

These signs disappear if the visceral cause improves. When such changes become chronic however, trophic alterations are noted, with increased thickening of the skin and subcutaneous tissue, and localised muscular contraction. Deep musculature may become hard, tense and hypersensitive. This may involve deep splinting contractions, involving two or more segments of the spine, with associated restriction of spinal motion. The costotransverse articulations may be significantly involved in such changes.

Patterns of somatic response will be found to differ from person to person, and to be unique, in terms of location, the number of segments involved, and whether or not the pattern is uni- or bilateral. The degree of intensity will also differ, and is related to the degree of acuteness of the visceral condition (Hix 1976). Research involving animals, as well as observations in humans, using regional nerve blocks, has helped to define site locations of response, in various forms of visceral dysfunction. Beal notes that three distinct groups of visceral involvement are found in respect of particular sites. These are:

1. T1–T5: heart and lungs
2. T5–T10: oesophagus, stomach, small intestine, liver, gall bladder, spleen, pancreas and adrenal cortex
3. T10–L2: large bowel, appendix, kidney, ureter, adrenal medulla, testes, ovaries, urinary bladder, prostate gland, uterus.

There appears to be a consensus as to sidedness being apparent, in reflexes of unpaired organs. Thus, left-sidedness is noted in conditions involving small intestine and the heart; right-sidedness for gall bladder disease and appendix. The stomach may produce reflex activity on either, or both sides. *Left side = the heart & small intestine* *Right side gallbladder disease appendix*

A number of studies have been concerned with the identification of such reflexes. One 5 year study involved over 5000 hospitalised patients (Kelso 1985). This concluded that most visceral disease appeared to influence more than one region, and that the number of spinal segments involved was related to the duration of the disease. Kelso noted in this study that there was an increase in the number of palpatory findings in the cervical region, related to patients with sinusitis, tonsillitis, diseases of the oesophagus and liver complaints. Soft tissue changes were noted in patients with gastritis, duodenal ulceration, pyelonephritis, chronic appendicitis and cholycystitis, in the region of T5–T12. *T5 - T12*

Palpating facilitated spinal tissues

Somatic dysfunction is assessed most usually by use of palpatory investigation and Beal (1983) insists that investigation should pay attention to the various soft tissue layers:

The skin for changes in texture, temperature and moisture; the subcutaneous tissue for changes in consistency and fluid; the superficial and deep musculature for tone, irritability, consistency, viscoelastic properties, and fluid content; and the deep fascial layers for textural changes.

He advises that, 'Special attention [should] be given to the examination of the costotransverse area, where it is felt that autonomic nerve effects are predominant,' and notes that tests for the quality and range of joints have not been found to differentiate between visceral reflexes and somatic changes, which confirms the importance of the soft tissue assessment in order to elicit such information.

Beal notes that the supine position is ideal for assessment of paraspinal tissues – the hand being gently inserted under the region, and pressure, or springing techniques applied (Fig. 3.4). He has not investigated the use of patient examination in the prone position, as he suggests that this position is precluded in acutely ill patients. Nevertheless, since Beal notes the difficulty of applying diagnostic measures with the patient supine when the mid to lower thoracic area is under review, a prone position is suggested, unless the patient cannot manage this. The

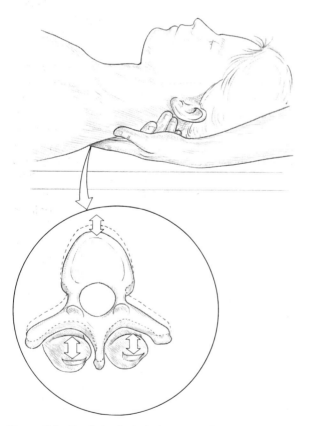

Figure 3.4 Beal's 'springing' assessment for paraspinal facilitation rigidity associated with segmental facilitation.

availability of a couch with a split head-piece would make this more comfortable. As we will see the methods employed by those using connective tissue massage involve the patient being seated. This helps in assessing skin and superficial tissue status, but is not really suitable for deeper penetration.

Beal suggests that the diagnosis of a paraspinal viscerosomatic reflex be based upon two or more adjacent spinal segments showing evidence of somatic dysfunction, and being located within the specific autonomic reflex area. There should be deep confluent spinal muscle splinting, and resistance to segmental joint motion. Skin and subcutaneous tissue changes which are consistent with the acuteness or chronicity of the reflex should be noted.

Specific identification of the origin of the reflex is, he suggests, difficult.

The usefulness of understanding the nature of such reflexes often involves clinical frustration, when, for instance, localised soft tissue dysfunction fails to respond to treatment. Suspicion may then be alerted to possible visceral activity maintaining the muscular or joint dysfunction.

According to Beal, treatment of the acute stage should be aimed primarily at breaking into the reflex arc. In cases of serious illness the treatment may consist of gentle digital pressure, of short duration, to affect a local change in superficial tissues. When relaxation has been accomplished in the subcutaneous and superficial paraspinal musculature, the deep muscle contraction can be addressed. The duration of treatment is dependent upon the patient's condition and perceived energy level. Beal suggests that acute conditions that are not life threatening may be addressed in a more aggressive manner (asthma is given as an example).

The authors suggest that NMT is also an ideal method of addressing soft tissue manifestations of such reflex activity, since NMT offers a diagnostic, as well as a therapeutic opportunity to address both superficial and deep tissues. Viscerosomatic reflex changes are just one of the many reasons for altered tissue findings, which may be noted in the general NMT assessment. Awareness of the possibility of what is being noted being of reflex origin adds to the potential for accurate diagnosis. In the following chapter a variety of other reflex systems are evaluated.

Causes of local facilitation

Melzack and Wall (1989) in their exhaustive investigation of pain, are clear in their statement that all chronic pain has myofascial trigger point activity as at least a part of its aetiology, and that in many instances trigger points are the major contributors to the pain.

A trigger point is a localised, palpable area of soft tissue which is painful on pressure and which refers symptoms, usually including pain, to a predictable target area some distance from itself. It is an area of local facilitation – which has developed following a very similar aetiological pathway to that occurring in segmental (spinal) facilitated areas.

Facilitation paraspinally and in general muscle tissue can be the result of repetitive minor or single major traumatic influences or stress factors (as described in Ch. 1). The form of facilitation which is our main focus in this chapter is a localised area of hyperirritability – the trigger point.

[handwritten: If pain is severe enough to seek professional help, pain is likely referred – the factor of trigger area involved]

Travell and Simons

Much research and clinical work has been done in recent years in this field by Janet Travell (Travell 1957, Travell & Simons 1986/93) who is on record as stating that if a pain is severe enough to cause a patient to seek professional advice (in the absence of organic disease) referred pain is likely to be a factor, and therefore a trigger area is probably involved. She maintains that patterns of referred pain are constant in distribution in all people, only the intensity of referred symptoms/pain will vary.

Among the effects of an active trigger point, apart from pain, there may be numbness, tingling, weakness, lack of normal range of movement. The aetiological myofascial trigger point for a particular pain pattern is always located in a particular part of a particular muscle (Webber 1973). While eradication of the trigger, by what-

ever appropriate means, can remove all symptoms, treatment of the target or reference area is useless.

TRIGGER POINTS

Trigger points are localised areas of deep tenderness and increased resistance and digital pressure on such a trigger will often produce twitching and fasciculation (see pp xiii–xv). Pressure maintained on such a point will produce referred pain in a predictable area. If there are a number of active trigger points the reference areas may overlap.

What is distinctive about active trigger points (myofascial trigger points) is that they also refer sensation or symptoms to a distinct target area, and that this target area is more or less reproducible in other individuals, when trigger points are located in similar positions. No other soft tissue dysfunction has this particular attribute.

Before an active trigger point exists there needs to be a period of evolution towards that unhappy state. This involves the development of soft tissue changes which would be palpable and probably sensitive or painful but which, until sufficient localised stress had been involved, would not refer symptoms onwards. In other words, most areas of sensitivity or pain which do not refer pain or other symptoms may be considered to be embryonic or evolutionary trigger points. A single trigger may refer pain to several reference sites and can give rise to embryonic, or satellite triggers. Travell describes, for example, how a trigger in the distal areas of the sternomastoid muscle can give rise to new triggers in the sternalis muscle, the pectoral muscle and/or serratus anterior (Travell 1981).

Travell's definition of a trigger point is that:

It lies in skeletal muscle, and is identified by localised deep tenderness, in a palpable firm band of muscle (muscle hardening); and at the point of maximum deep hyperalgesia, by a positive 'jump sign', a visible shortening of the part of the muscle which contains the band. To elicit the jump sign most effectively, one must place the relaxed muscle under moderate passive tension, and snap the band briskly with the palpating finger.

[handwritten: 80% of Major trigger points are on established acupuncture points]

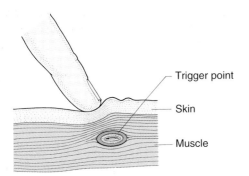

Figure 3.5 Trigger points are areas of local facilitation which can be housed in any soft tissue structure, most usually muscle and/or fascia. Palpation from the skin or at depth may be required to localise these.

The trigger point must also refer symptoms or sensations to a target area. Otherwise, rather than being active, it may be a latent trigger point, which could be activated by stress or strain on the tissues in which it lies. The difference between most other areas of discrete palpable soft tissue dysfunction and an active trigger, is this quality of referring symptoms. All other points may be prospective triggers, but are not active (Fig. 3.5).

The causes of trigger point presence can relate to any combination of physical or psychic stress factors which result in alterations in normal tone in muscles, fascia and other soft tissues which,

in turn, can effect changes in joint play, breathing, posture etc. The progression from hypertonicity through retained metabolic wastes and relative ischaemia, in muscle so affected, has been discussed previously (p. 6). The feature of ischaemia and prolonged stress seems to be a major predisposing condition in the production of trigger points and their referred pain and dysfunction. Travell's research has shown that a series of embryonic trigger points develop in target/referred areas so that in time a chain reaction of triggers can exist.

The pathways which allow particular triggers to produce symptoms in target areas do not follow known neurological patterns, nor do they precisely mimic the pathways of traditional Chinese medicine meridians – although there is some overlap. Melzack has shown that roughly 80% of major trigger point sites are on established acupuncture points (Wall & Melzack 1989).

Travell and Simons have stated:

> In the core of the trigger lies a muscle spindle which is in trouble for some reason. Visualise a spindle like a strand of yarn in a knitted sweater . . . a metabolic crisis takes place which increases the temperature locally in the trigger point, shortens a minute part of the muscle (sarcomere) – like a snag in a sweater, and reduces the supply of oxygen and nutrients into the trigger point. During this disturbed episode an influx of calcium occurs and the muscle spindle does not

[handwritten: description of trigger point]

[handwritten: causes]

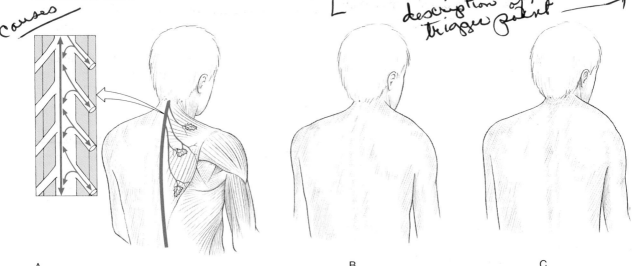

Figure 3.6A,B,C Trigger points evolve in specific areas of stressed myofascial tissue. As these tissues compensate progressively towards an ever more dysfunctional fibrotic state, so does the activity of associated trigger points increase.

[handwritten annotations: "Point of trigger - lack of oxygen in spot. Calcium building in cell of muscle spindle - can't relax"]

have enough energy to pump the calcium outside the cell where it belongs. Thus a vicious cycle is maintained and the muscle spindle can't seem to loosen up and the affected muscle can't relax. (Fig. 3.6)

Simons has reviewed the work of others who have tested this concept and found that at the centre of the trigger points there is indeed a lack of oxygen compared with that existing in the muscles which surround it (Simons 1994).

Travell (Travell & Simons 1983/92) has confirmed that the following factors can all help to maintain and enhance trigger point activity:

- Nutritional deficiency, especially vitamins C, B-complex and iron
- Hormonal imbalances (low thyroid hormone production, menopausal or premenstrual situations)
- Infections (bacteria, viruses or yeast)
- Allergies (wheat and dairy in particular)
- Low oxygenation of tissues (aggravated by tension, stress, inactivity, poor respiration).

A number of methods exist for the obliteration of such trigger points, ranging from use of pharmacological agents such as novocaine or xylocain, to coolant sprays and acupuncture techniques. It is noteworthy that direct digital pressure techniques can also effectively deactivate, trigger points – if only temporarily in many instances. Clinical experience has shown that an absolute requirement for trigger point deactivation (apart from removal of the causes) involves the need to restore the muscle in which the trigger lies to its normal resting length.

A failure to achieve this goal means that all other methods of treating trigger points are likely to provide only short-term relief. It is vital to remember that a trigger point is self-perpetuating unless it is correctly and sufficiently treated. This means that, once symptoms have been relieved, the muscle containing the trigger must be gently stretched to its longest resting length. Failing this, symptoms will return, irrespective of the technique used (chilling, pressure, injection, acupuncture etc.). Such stretching should be gradual and gentle and the recommendation of Lewit, Travell and Simons is that muscle energy technique (MET), in which

gentle isometric contractions followed by stretch are employed, is the method of choice to achieve that stretching (Lewit 1991, Travell & Simons 1992). Lewit suggests that, in many instances, stretching is adequate in itself in deactivating trigger point activity.

Other views on trigger points

[handwritten annotation: "Stretching !!! must be done following any kind of treatment"]

In order to gain further understanding of the significance of these widespread noxious entities, it is essential to be aware of the process of facilitation, as well as Selye's general and local adaptation syndromes (see Ch. 1, p. 5 and Ch. 10 on clinical applications of NMT). We need, also, to be aware of views of others who have tried to make sense of the myriad systems which have identified patterns of reflex activity in surface tissues (as discussed in the following chapter, p. 43).

Mennell

Mennell (1975) agrees that a muscle that can attain and maintain its normal resting length is a pain-free muscle. One that cannot (a muscle in spasm) is usually a source of pain, regardless of whether the source of the spasm is in that muscle or not. Whatever the means used to 'block' the trigger activity, and whatever the neuropathological routes involved, the critical factor in the restoration of pain-free normality is that, during any relief from the state of spasm or contraction, the affected muscle should have its normal resting length restored by stretching. Mennell defines trigger points as localised palpable spots of deep hypersensitivity from which noxious impulses bombard the CNS to give rise to referred pain. Mennell favours chilling the trigger area by vapocoolant or ice-massage – an approach supported by Travell and Simons, who now both advocate MET as well. Details of their recommended methods will be given in the treatment section (p. 110).

[handwritten annotation: "chilling the trigger area or ice-massage"]

Chaitow

Chaitow has proposed that a sequence of treatment to achieve trigger point deactivation –

commencing with palpation/identification utilising NMT, followed by ischaemic compression (also NMT), followed by adoption of a positional release posture (such as is used in osteopathic functional technique or strain/counterstrain) – should be followed by a stretching of the tissues housing the trigger point. The stretching in this sequence can follow a focused (to activate the fibres involved) isometric contraction, or be applied at the same time as the contraction – introducing an isolytic muscle energy approach into the methodology.

This sequence has been dubbed integrated neuromuscular inhibition technique (INIT) and will be elaborated on in the chapters dealing with treatment (Chaitow 1994).

PATHOPHYSIOLOGY OF FIBROMYALGIA/FIBROSITIS/ MYODYSNEURIA

The changes which occur in tissue involved in the onset of myodysneuria/fibromyalgia, according to Gutstein, are thought to be initiated by localised sympathetic predominance, associated with changes in the hydrogen ion concentration and calcium and sodium balance in the tissue fluids (Petersen 1934). This is associated with vasoconstriction and hypoxia/ischaemia. Pain results, it is thought, from these alterations affecting the pain sensors and proprioceptors. Muscle spasm and hard nodular localised tetanic contractions of muscle bundles (Bayer 1950), together with vasomotor and musculomotor stimulation, intensify each other, creating a vicious cycle of self-perpetuating impulses. There are varied and complex patterns of referred symptoms which may result from such 'trigger' areas, as well as local pain and minor disturbances.

Such sensations as aching, soreness, tenderness, heaviness and tiredness may all be manifest, as may modification of muscular activity due to contraction resulting in tightness, stiffness, swelling etc.

Recent research has resulted in strict guidelines for a diagnosis of fibromyalgia from the American College of Rheumatology (Wolfe 1990):

1. History of widespread pain.

Pain is considered widespread when all of the following are present: pain in the left side of the body, pain in the right side of the body, pain above the waist and pain below the waist. In addition there should be pain in the spine or the neck or front of the chest, or thoracic spine or low back.

2. Pain in 11 of 18 palpated tender point sites.

There should be pain on pressure (around 4 kg of pressure maximum) on not less than 11 of the following sites (Fig. 3.7):

- Either side of the base of the skull where the suboccipital muscles insert
- Either side of the side of the neck between the 5th and 7th cervical vertebra – technically described as between the 'anterior aspects of inter-transverse spaces'
- Either side of the body on the midpoint of the muscle which runs from the neck to the shoulder (upper trapezius)
- Either side of the body on the origin of the supraspinatus muscle which runs along the upper border of the shoulder blade
- Either side, on the upper surface of the rib, where the 2nd rib meets the breast bone, in the pectoral muscle
- On the outer aspect of either elbow just below the prominence (epicondyle)
- In the large buttock muscles, either side, on the upper outer aspect in the fold in front of the muscle (gluteus medius)
- Just behind the large prominence of either hip joint in the muscular insertion of piriformis muscle
- On either knee in the fatty pad just above the inner aspect of the joint.

A puzzle

The question is often asked – is fibromyalgia the same as myofascial pain syndrome (pain problems in which trigger points are clearly involved)?

Do trigger points actually cause fibromyalgia?

A condition called myofascial pain syndrome (MPS) – a disorder in which pain of a persistent aching type is referred to a number of target areas by triggers lying some distance away – has

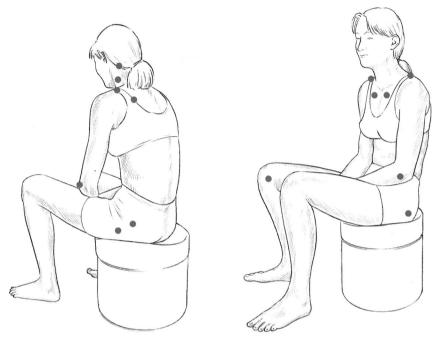

Figure 3.7   The sites of the 18 fibromyalgia tender points as defined by the American College of Rheumatologists.

long been recognised as a cause of severe and chronic pain. Since many experts insist that the 'tender' points which are palpated when diagnosing fibromyalgia need to refer pain elsewhere if they are to be taken seriously in the diagnosis (making them trigger points by definition) the question needs to be asked whether MPS is not the self-same thing as FMS?

The answer is – not quite.

Scandinavian researchers showed in 1986 that around 65% of people with fibromyalgia had identifiable trigger points, and it is clear, therefore, that there is an overlap between FMS and MPS.

D. P. Baldry, a leading British physician/acupuncturist, has summarised the similarities and differences between these two conditions (Baldry 1993) as follows: *Both f myoalgia and myofascial pain*

The two conditions are *similar* or identical in that both fibromyalgia and myofascial pain syndrome: *alike*

- Are affected by cold weather
- May involve increased sympathetic nerve

activity and may involve conditions such as Raynaud's phenomenon
- Have tension headaches and paraesthesia as a major associated symptom
- Are unaffected by anti-inflammatory pain-killing medication whether of the cortisone type or standard formulations.

Fibromyalgia and myofascial pain syndrome (MPS) are *different* in that: *Different*

- MPS affects males and females equally, fibromyalgia mainly (80%) females
- MPS is usually local to an area such as the neck and shoulders, or low back and legs, although it can affect a number of parts of the body at the same time, whereas fibromyalgia is a generalised problem – often involving all four 'corners' of the body at the same time
- Muscles which contain areas which feel 'like a tight rubber band' are found in the muscles of around 30% of people with MPS but more than 60% of people with FMS
- People with FMS have poorer muscle endurance than people with MPS

- MPS can sometimes be bad enough to cause disturbed sleep, whereas in fibromyalgia the sleep disturbance has a more causative role, and is a pronounced feature of the condition
- MPS produces no morning stiffness whereas fibromyalgia does
- There is not usually fatigue associated with MPS, while it is common in fibromyalgia
- MPS can sometimes lead to depression (reactive) and anxiety whereas, in a small percentage of fibromyalgia cases, these conditions can be the trigger for the start of the condition
- Conditions such as irritable bowel syndrome, dysmenorrhoea and a feeling of swollen joints are noted in fibromyalgia but seldom in MPS
- Low dosage tricyclic antidepressant drugs are helpful in dealing with the sleep problems, and many of the symptoms, of fibromyalgia – but not of MPS
- Exercise programmes (cardiovascular fitness) can help some fibromyalgia patients, according to experts, but this is not a useful approach in MPS
- The outlook for people with MPS is excellent since the trigger points usually respond quickly to massage, manipulative or acupuncture techniques, whereas the outlook for fibromyalgia is less positive – with a lengthy treatment and recovery phase being the norm.

Conclusion and hypothesis

We have seen how hyperreactive local (trigger point) and spinal areas can arise and be maintained and/or aggravated as a result of repetitive and continuous stress of one sort or another.

What we see in fibromyalgia is that areas of the brain behave in a facilitated manner – and that this hyperreactive brain activity could well be another version of this same phenomenon (facilitation). If so, we can learn much about fibromyalgia from our experience of handling localised facilitation processes such as trigger points.

Korr's studies discussed previously (p. 31) show that facilitated areas act as 'neurological lenses' – focusing whatever stress impacts on the person as a whole through these sensitised tissues.

If that 'tissue' happens to be (a part of) the brain, we have a situation in which it becomes imperative for stress of all sorts (climatic, emotional, structural/postural, nutritional, toxic, infection, allergy, etc. etc.) to be minimised, and this includes tailoring therapeutic interventions to be as non-invasive as possible (deep massage causes increased muscle pain in fibromyalgia whereas light massage does not).

Constitutional therapeutic approaches such as deep relaxation, non-stressful hydrotherapy, wellness massage and similar methods are more likely to be helpful than anything which makes adaptive demands on an already compromised individual.

Summary. Trigger points are certainly often part – in some cases the major part – of the pain suffered by people with fibromyalgia. When they are present (as they certainly are if pressure on the 'tender point' produces pain somewhere else in the body) – we need to know more about them and how they can be successfully treated.

In the next chapter an overview will be presented of other reflex systems, awareness of which should add to our comprehensive understanding of myofascial trigger points.

REFERENCES

Baldry P 1993 Acupuncture trigger points and musculoskeletal pain. Churchill Livingstone, Edinburgh

Bayer H 1950 Pathophysiology of muscular rheumatism. Zeitschrift für Raeumaforschung 9: 210

Beal M 1983 Palpatory testing of somatic dysfunction in patients with cardiovascular disease. Journal of the American Osteopathic Association July

Beal M 1985 Viscerosomatic reflexes: a review. Journal of the American Osteopathic Association 85(12): 786–801

Brugger A 1962 Pseudoradikulare syndrome. Acta Rheumatol 19: 1

Chaitow L 1994 Integrated neuro-muscular inhibition technique in treatment of pain and trigger points. British Osteopathic Journal XIII: 17–21

Cornelius A 1909 Die neurenpunkt lehre, vol 2. George Thins, Leipzig

Denslow J, Korr I et al 1949 Quantitative studies of chronic facilitation. American Journal of Physiology 150: 229–238

Dittrich R J 1954 Somatic pain and autonomic concomitants. American Journal of Surgery

Dowling D 1991 In: DiGiovanna E (ed.) An osteopathic approach to diagnosis and treatment. Lippincott, Philadelphia

Dvorak J, Dvorak V 1984 Manual medicine diagnostics. Georg Thieme Verlag, Stuttgart

Dubs R 1950 Beitrag zur anatomie der lumbosakralen region. Fortschritte der Neurologie – Psychiatrie 18: 69

Evans J Reflex sympathetic dystrophy. Annals of Internal Medicine

Feinstein B, Longton J, Jameson R, Schiller F 1954 Experiments on pain referred from deep somatic tissues. Journal of Bone and Joint Surgery 36A: 981

Gutstein R 1944 A review of myodysneuria (fibrositis). American Practitioner and Digest of Treatments 6(4): 114–124

Gutstein R 1944 The role of abdominal fibrositis in functional indigestion. Mississippi Valley Medical Journal 66: 114–124

Gutstein R 1956 The role of craniocervical myodysneuria in functional ocular disorders. American Practitioner's Digest of Treatments November

Hix E 1976 Reflex viscerosomatic reference phenomena. Osteopathic Annals 4(12): 496–503

Hockaday J, Whitty 1967 Patterns of referred pain in normal subjects. Brain 90: 481

Kellgren J 1938 Observations on referred pain coming from muscle. Clinical Science 3: 175–190

Kellgren J 1939 On the distribution of pain arising from deep somatic structures. Clinical Science 4: 35–46

Kelso 1985 Viscerosomatic reflexes: a review. Journal of the American Osteopathic Association 85(12): 786–801

Korr I 1970 Physiological basis of osteopathic medicine.

Postgraduate Institute of Osteopathic Medicine and Surgery, New York

Korr I 1975 Proprioceptors and somatic dysfuncion. Journal of the American Osteopathic Association 74: 638

Korr I 1976 Spinal cord as organiser of disease process. Academy of Applied Osteopathy Yearbook 1976

Korr I (ed.) 1977 Neurobiological mechanisms in manipulation. Plenum Press, New York

Korr I 1986 Somatic dysfunction. Journal of the American Osteopathic Association 86(2): 109–114

Lewis T 1938 Suggestions relating to the study of somatic pain. BMJ 1: 321–325

Lewit K 1991 Manipulation in rehabilitation of the locomotor system. Butterworths, London

Lewit K 1992 Manipulative therapy in rehabilitation of the locomotor system. Butterworths, London

Mennell J 1975 The therapeutic use of cold. Journal of the American Osteopathic Association 74 August

Patterson M 1976 Model mechanism for spinal segmental facilitation. Academy of Applied Osteopathy Yearbook 1976

Petersen W 1934 The patient and the weather: autonomic disintegration. Edward Bros, Ann Arbor

Simons D 1994 Myofascial pain syndromes. Journal of Musculoskeletal Pain 2(2): 113–121

Speransky A 1943 A basis for the theory of medicine. International Publishers, New York

Sutter M 1975 Versuch einer Wesensbestimmung pseudoradikularer syndrome. Schweizerische Rundschau für Medizin Praxis 63: 42

Travell J 1957 Symposium on mechanism and management of pain syndromes. Proc Rudolph Virchow Medical Soc

Travell J 1981 Identification of myofascial trigger point syndromes. Archives of Physical Medicine 62: 100

Travell J, Bigelow N 1947 Role of somatic trigger areas in the patterns of hysteria. Psychosomatic Medicine 9(6): 353–363

Travell J, Simons D 1983 Myofascial pain and dysfunction (vol 1) The trigger point manual. Williams and Wilkins

Travell J, Simons D 1992 Myofascial pain and dysfunction (vol 2) The trigger point manual. Williams and Wilkins

Wall P, Melzack R 1989 Textbook of pain. Churchill Livingstone, Edinburgh

Webber T D 1973 Diagnosis and modification of headache and shoulder, arm, hand syndromes. Journal of the American Osteopathic Association 72 March

Wolfe F et al 1990 American College of Rheumatology 1990 criteria for classification of fibromyalgia. Arthritis and Rheumatism 33: 160–172

Wolfe F, Simons D 1992 Fibromyalgia and myofascial pain syndromes. Journal of Rheumatology 19(6): 944–951

4

The variety of reflex points

IDENTIFIED REFLEX AREAS

In this chapter some of the major systems which have identified and classified reflex areas on the body surface will be discussed, since many of the 'points' which these identify are bound to be accessed during the application of NMT in an assessment or a treatment mode.

Osteopathic physician Eileen DiGiovanna (1991) states, 'Today many physicians believe there is a relationship among trigger points, acupuncture points and Chapman's reflexes. Precisely what the relationship may be is unknown.'

She quotes from a prestigious osteopathic pioneer, George Northup, who stated as far back as 1941:

One cannot escape the feelings that all of the seemingly diverse observations (regarding reflex patterns) are but views of the same iceberg the tip of which we are beginning to see, without understanding either its magnitude or its depth of importance (Northup 1941).

Awareness of the reflex potential of the body surface widens the therapeutic potential of NMT, although deciding which of the many possible applications of reflex activity to utilise in diagnosis or treatment can be a daunting task. The discussion in this text of these reflex systems and classifications should not be taken as indicating recommendation for their use, merely recognition of the fact that they are widely used, and that NMT offers an additional means of access and employment of their potential.

Felix Mann, one of the pioneers of acupuncture in the West, has entered the controversy as to the existence, or otherwise, of acupuncture meridians (and indeed acupuncture points). At a conference in New York in 1983, Mann, in an effort to alter the emphasis which traditional acupuncture places on the specific charted positions of points, stated (Mann 1983):

McBurney's point, in appendicitis, has a defined position. In reality it may be 10 cms higher, lower, to the left or right. It may be one centimetre in diameter, or occupy the whole of the abdomen, or not occur at all. Acupuncture points are often the same, and hence it is pointless to speak of acupuncture points in the classical traditional way. Carefully performed electrical resistance measurements do not show alterations in the skin resistance to electricity, corresponding with classical acupuncture points. There are so many acupuncture points mentioned in some modern books, that there is no skin left which is not an acupuncture point. In cardiac disease, pain and tenderness may occur in the arm however this does not occur more frequently along the course of the heart meridian, than anywhere else in the arm.

Hence, Mann concludes, meridians do not exist, or – more confusingly perhaps – that the whole body is an acupuncture point!

Leaving aside the validity of Mann's comment, it is true to say that if all the multitude of points described in acupuncture, traditional and modern, together with those points described by Travell and co-workers, Chapman, Jones, Bennett (see later in this chapter, p. 53), were to be placed together on one map of the body surface, we would soon come to the conclusion that the entire body surface is a 'potential acupuncture point'. This realisation is supported by Speransky's findings from the 1930s, as discussed in Chapter 3 (p. 26).

Are all tender points trigger points?

A number of respected researchers and clinicians are frequently in error when they describe localised soft tissue areas which palpate as sensitive but which do not refer symptoms elsewhere, as trigger points. Certainly a trigger point will always be palpable, and will always be sensitive to pressure, but then so will most other 'points', whether these be Chapman's reflexes, Gutstein's myodysneuria points, Jones's tender points or acupuncture alarm points. These, however, will not necessarily refer painful symptoms to distant sites in the obvious manner displayed by trigger points. This is not to say that any 'tender' or sensitive point cannot become a trigger point, since clearly, before it is active, a trigger point has to evolve and in its earlier stages will be painful, sensitive or tender, but may at the time of palpation not be sufficiently sensitised and hyperreactive to refer pain and other symptoms. If a point 'belonging' to any of the various classifications discussed below do refer symptoms in the manner of trigger points, then they can be so classified and treated.

Some of the major 'point' classifications involving reflex activity and with a diagnostic potential are considered in this chapter in alphabetical order (not in order of apparent importance).

ACUPUNCTURE POINTS

Soft tissue changes often produce organised discrete areas which act as generators of secondary

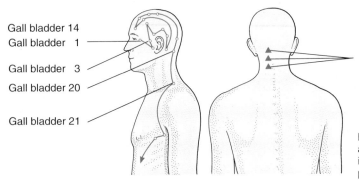

Gall bladder 14
Gall bladder 1
Gall bladder 3
Gall bladder 20
Gall bladder 21

Common trigger point sites on the Bladder meridian

Figure 4.1A,B The location of some important acupuncture points on the head and neck. Research indicates that over 75% of defined acupuncture points are also sites of common trigger points.

problems. It would be advantageous to examine briefly another aspect of 'trigger' points: that is, the existence of a network of points which is supposedly constantly capable of reflex activity. This network is, of course, the pattern of acupuncture points (Fig. 4.1). What is of interest is that the location of these fixed anatomical points is capable of corroboration by electrical detection, each point being evidenced by a small area of lowered electrical resistance.

When 'active', due presumably to reflex stimulation, these points become even more detectable, as the electrical resistance lowers further. The skin overlying them also alters and becomes hyperalgesic and not difficult to palpate as differing from surrounding skin. Active acupuncture points also become sensitive to pressure and this is of value to the therapist since the finding of sensitive areas during palpation or treatment is of diagnostic importance. Sensitive and painful areas that do not have detectable tissue changes as part of their make up may well be 'active' acupuncture points (or *Tsubo*, which means 'points on the human body' in Japanese). Not only are these points detectable and sensitive, but they are also amenable to treatment by direct pressure techniques. They are, therefore, well worth studying.

One of the leading Oriental experts on pressure techniques is Katsusuke Serizawe, who discusses a 'nerve-reflex' theory for the existence of these points (Serizawe 1980):

The nerve reflex theory holds that, when an abnormal condition occurs in an internal organ, alterations take place in the skin and muscles related to that organ by means of the nervous system. These alterations occur as reflex actions. The nervous system, extending throughout the internal organs, like the skin, the subcutaneous tissues, and the muscles, constantly transmits information about the physical condition to the spinal cord and the brain. These information impulses, which are centripetal in nature, set up a reflex action that causes symptoms of the internal organic disorder to manifest themselves in the surface areas of the body. The reflex symptoms may be classified into the following three major groups: (a) sensation reflexes; (b) interlocking reflexes; (c) autonomic system reflexes.

(a) Sensation reflexes. When an abnormal centripetal impulse travels to the spinal cord, reflex action causes the skin at the spinal column affected by the impulse to become hypersensitive. This sensitivity to pain is especially notable in the skin, subcutaneous tissues, and muscles located close to the surface, since these organs are richly supplied with sensory nerves.

(b) Interlocked reflexes. An abnormality in an internal organ causes a limited contraction, stiffening, or lumping of the muscles in the area near the part of the body that is connected by means of nerves to the affected organ. Stiffness in the shoulders, back, arms, and legs are symptoms of this kind. In effect, the interlocked reflex actions amount to a hardening and stiffening of the muscles to protect the ailing internal organ from excess stimulus. When the abnormality in the organ is grave, however, the stiffening of the muscles is not limited to a small area, but extends over large parts of the body.

(c) Autonomic system reflexes. Abnormalities in the internal organs sometimes set up reflex action in the sweat glands, the sebaceous glands, the pilomotor muscles, and the blood vessels in the skin. The reflex action may cause excess sweat or drying of the skin as the consequence of cessation of sweat secretion. Its effect on the pilomotor muscles may be to cause the condition known as goose flesh. The sebaceous glands may be stimulated to secrete excess sebum, thus causing abnormal oiliness in the skin; or they may stop secreting sebum, thus making the skin abnormally dry. The reflex action may cause chills or flushing because of its effects on the blood vessels in the skin.

I have discussed the ways in which abnormalities in internal organs cause changes in the conditions of the surface organs of the body however the intimate relation between internal organs and external ones has a reverse effect as well; that is, stimulation to the skin and muscles affects the condition of the internal organs and tissues. For instance, stimulation transmitted to the spinal cord from the body surface sets up a reflex action in the internal organ that is controlled by the nerves at the level of the spinal column receiving external stimuli. Stimuli of this kind instigate peristaltic motion or contraction in the organ. The effect of such external stimulation on blood vessels and on the secretion of hormones has been scientifically verified.

The reader will note a conceptual link between the forces underlying Tsubo usage and our understanding of facilitation as explained in Chapter 3 (p. 30).

Quite obviously, there may be more effective ways of dealing with organ dysfunction than by pressure techniques to Tsubo/acupuncture points. However, since our study is concerned basically with manual treatment, it is worth taking account of the knowledge accumulated by the Chinese and Japanese over many centuries.

Acupuncture points and their morphology

Melzack, and other researchers, maintain that there is little, if any, difference between acupuncture points and most trigger points (Wall & Melzack 1989, Travell & Simons 1992) and since all sensitive points are capable of becoming trigger points, any research into the structure of acupuncture points should enhance our understanding of trigger point activity.

The morphology of acupuncture points has been studied, notably by Jean Bosey (1984), Professor of Anatomy at Montpellier University, France. Some of his major conclusions, in summary, are as follows:

Points are situated in palpable depressions ('cupules'). The skin (epiderm) over the point is a little thinner at the cupule level, under which lies a fibrous cone in which there is frequently found either a neurovascular formation, or simply a cutaneous neurovascular bundle. Free nerve endings are noted, and the presence, beneath the point, of Golgi endings and Pacini corpuscles is common. Connective tissues lie below at varying depths. Fascia and aponeurosis are noted and, it is stated: 'A passage of vessels and nerves, through the fascia, is very often found under the acupuncture point.'

An anatomical study of 100 acupuncture points showed that they overlay large nerve trunks in 42% of cases, large veins in 40% and cutaneous neurovascular pedicals in 18%. The effect, in deeper structures, of stimulation (by needling or pressure) of muscle and tendon receptors, is noted, but this is thought to be indirect, rather than direct, because of the extremely small size of, for example, muscle spindles and Golgi tendon organs. The practice of manipulating the needle, thus imposing a degree of traction on the underlying (muscular) tissue, is noted, and this would, it is observed, impose stimulation on such receptor organs. Fat is also a common factor in the morphology of points, and this, and the connective tissue, are thought to be key factors in the achievement of the 'acupuncture sensation' which accompanies successful treatment. The conclusion reached is that a number of tissues are simultaneously affected by any particular acupuncture needle (and, the author stresses, by strong finger pressure).

Some points, when dissected, showed that neurovascular structures lie immediately below the point, which could account for the particular effects noted by such points being treated. This is of interest to those using Bennett's neurovascular points. The implications for those practitioners not employing needles, and who rely on pressure techniques in order to provide stimulus or sedation to such areas, is that, if accurately applied, the effects of pressure should be identical (to needle acupuncture), especially in relation to pain control.

Acupuncture and applied kinesiology (AK)

An attempt to correlate the various reflex systems and methods has been made by the American chiropractor Dr George Goodheart. His system of applied kinesiology involves testing muscle groups for weaknesses and then, depending upon the results of such tests, using various massage and pressure techniques applied to specific locations (points) in order to normalise function. These points correspond to Chapman's reflexes, acupuncture points and other less well known reflex systems. Many of Goodheart's techniques, theories and methods support and utilise methods that are in line with neuromuscular technique, and these will be mentioned in the treatment section (p. 87).

Acupressure and pain thresholds

It has been shown that pain thresholds can be dramatically elevated by pressure techniques applied to specific points. Researchers at the Peking Medical College conducted complex experiments which demonstrated that finger pressure acupuncture caused a rise of 133% in pain threshold of rabbits (using radiant heat as the painful stimulus). When cerebrospinal fluid was perfused from one rabbit to another after such experiments, the recipient rabbit was found to have achieved a rise in pain threshold of up to

80%. This suggested the presence of hormone-like substances produced by the brain in response to the original acupressure stimulus. These substances are now known to be enkephalins and endorphins, and these play a role in NMT pain control. The point used in these tests was equivalent to the acupuncture point known as Bladder 60, posterior to the ankle (externally) and just anterior to the Achilles tendon.

Acupuncture points and trigger points: are they the same phenomenon?

Since they spatially occupy the same positions in at least 70% of cases (Wall & Melzack 1989) there is often a coincidence of treatment in that a trigger point could be 'mistaken' for an active acupuncture point and vice versa. Melzack and Wall have concluded that, 'trigger points and acupuncture points when used for pain control, though discovered independently and labelled differently, represent the same phenomenon'.

Baldry (1993) does not agree however, claiming differences in their structural makeup. He states:

It would seem likely that they are of two different types, and their close spatial correlation is because there are A-delta afferent-innervated [fast transmitting receptors with a high threshold and sensitive to sharply pointed stimuli or heat produced stimulation] acupuncture points in the skin and subcutaneous tissues immediately above the intramuscularly placed, predominantly C afferent-innervated [slow transmitting, low threshold, widely distributed and sensitive to chemicals – such as those released by damaged cells – mechanical or thermal stimulus] trigger points.

Clearly, stimulation of an area which has, beneath the contacting instrument or digit, both an acupuncture and a trigger point, will influence both types of neural transmission and both 'points'. Which route of reflex stimulation is producing a therapeutic effect, or whether other mechanisms altogether are at work – endorphin release for example – is therefore open to debate. This debate can be further widened if we include the vast array of other reflex influences identified by other systems and workers as discussed later in this chapter (p. 51).

Whereas traditional Oriental concepts focus on 'energy' imbalances in reaction to acupuncture points, there exist also a number of Western interpretations.

Melzack, Stillwell and Fox (Melzack et al 1977) have assumed that acupuncture points represent areas of abnormal physiological activity, producing a continuous, low-level input into the CNS. They suggested that this might eventually lead to a combining with noxious stimuli deriving from other structures, innervated by the same segments, to produce an increased awareness of pain and distress. They found it reasonable to assume that trigger points and acupuncture points represented the same phenomenon, having found that the location of trigger points on Western maps, and acupuncture points used commonly in painful conditions, showed a remarkable 70% correlation in position.

It is interesting that the link between the source of pain or tender points, and the referred area of pain noted in trigger points, in many instances seems to travel along the routes of traditional acupuncture meridians, but certainly not always. Spontaneous pain in such a point, according to acupuncture tradition, indicates the need for urgent attention. It is not the intention of this book to provide instruction in acupuncture methodology, nor to necessarily endorse the views expressed by traditional acupuncture in relation to meridians and their purported connection with organs and systems. However, it would be shortsighted to ignore the accumulated wisdom which has led many thousands of skilled practitioners to ascribe particular roles to these points (for example Alarm, Associated and Akabane, see p. 49). As far as a manual therapy is concerned, there seems to be value in having awareness of the reported roles of particular acupuncture points, and of incorporating this into diagnostic and therapeutic settings.

As we palpate and search through the soft tissues, in basic neuromuscular technique, we are bound to come across areas of sensitivity which relate to these points. They are also often found to overlap with neurolymphatic and neurovascular points, as described elsewhere in this text.

For example, reflex number 19 in Chapman's reflexes, which relates to the urethra, is identical to the neurovascular point of the bladder, and the acupuncture alarm point of the Bladder meridian. Careful comparison will show many such overlaps. General guidance as to how to treat acupuncture points, which are sensitive, must relate to whether a stimulating or sedating effect is desired. The body often seems to utilise therapeutic stimulation to its best advantage. Selye has shown us (see Chapter 1, p. 5) that homoeostatic mechanisms are at work, so that any stimulus, if appropriate and not excessive, can result in a beneficial response. In accord with the methods used in treating neurolymphatic and neurovascular points (described elsewhere in this chapter, p. 51–53) it is suggested that, to some extent, the 'feel' of the tissues be allowed to guide the operator. A change (in the sense of a release of tension, or a softening, or a sensing of a gentle pulsation in the tissues) is often an indication of an adequate degree of therapy. In order to sedate what is an overactive point, up to 5 minutes of sustained or intermittent pressure, or rotary contact, may be required.

For stimulation, the timing could involve between 20 seconds and 2 minutes. By this time some degree of change should be palpable. As must be clear, if pressure is sustained beyond a certain point quite the opposite effect will be achieved. This is a common natural phenomenon which occurs in response to all factors in life, which are initially stimulating. If prolonged, they become enervating or exhausting, and in terms of therapy this is undesirable unless anaesthesia is required.

A short cold (water) application for example will stimulate, whereas a long one will sedate, and too much can kill. The words of Speransky and Selye should be recalled (p. 5 & p. 26), and the minimum effort used, consistent with achieving a response.

We have previously noted that many of the different reflex systems have points which seem to be interchangeable, and that many of these are traditional acupuncture points. In terms of local pain, the view of Chifuyu Takeshige (Takeshige 1985), Professor of Physiology at Showa University, is that: 'The acupuncture point of treatment of muscle pain is the pain-producing muscle itself.'

Respected acupuncture clinicians, such as George Ulett suggest that, 'acupuncture points are nothing more than time honoured muscle motor points'. Professor C. Chan Gunn, however, finds this too simple an explanation, and states: 'Calling acupuncture points "motor points" or "myofascial trigger points" is too simple. They are Golgi tendon organs.' These, and other researchers, are quoted by Stephen Botek, Assistant Professor of Clinical Psychiatry, New York Medical College (Ernst 1983). He believes that 'myofascial needling', is the term of choice to define that type of acupuncture which dispenses with traditional explanations as to acupuncture's effects. The points utilised in a specific study (Botek 1985) were Large Intestine 4 (Hoku) in the web between thumb and the first finger; and Stomach 36 (Tsu san li) below the knee. The study recorded skin temperature of the face, hands and feet. It was found that, as compared to a resting period, both manual and electrical stimulation of both points induced a general warming effect. This was immediate in the face (Lewith & Kenyon 1984), and appeared after 10 to 15 minutes in hands and feet. The temperature increase was notably more marked after manual acupressure than after electrical stimulation. Manual stimulation of these points was shown to be more effective than other forms of stimulation.

George Lewith and Julian Kenyon (1984) point to a variety of suggestions having been made as to the mechanisms via which acupuncture, or acupressure, achieve their pain relieving results. These include neurological explanations such as the 'gate control theory'. This, and variations on this theme, look at the various structures of the central nervous system and the brain in order to define the precise mechanisms involved in acupuncture's pain relieving action.

This in itself is seen to be an incomplete explanation, and humoral (endorphin release etc.) and psychological factors are also shown to be involved in modifying the patient's perception of pain.

A combination of reflex and direct neurological elements, as well as the involvement of a variety of secretions, such as enkephalins and endorphins, are thought to be the modus operandi of acupressure, and probably of all of the various systems of reflex activity discussed in this section (neurolymphatics etc.).

Many of the points of referred pain and tenderness used in Western medical diagnosis are also acupuncture points, for example:

- Head's zones could be shown to include most acupuncture points, especially the Alarm and Associated points (given below).
- The points noted as being 'tender' in appendicitis, such as McBurney's, Clado's, Cope's, Kummel's, Lavitas', are on the Stomach, Spleen and Kidney meridians of traditional acupuncture, and these are used by acupuncturists in treating appendicitis.
- Gastric ulcer patients produce tenderness at a site known as Boas' point, and this is sited precisely on Bladder point 21, which is the Associated point of the Stomach meridian.
- Brewer's point, in Western medicine, is noted in kidney infection, and this is Bladder point 20, the Associated point for the Spleen (in traditional acupuncture this has a controlling role over water, the element of the kidneys).

The degree of overlap between these well known points can also be noted when comparing other classification systems of points.

Ah Shi points

Acupuncture methodology also includes the treatment of points which are not listed on the meridian maps, and which are known as Ah Shi points. These include all painful points which arise spontaneously, usually in relation to particular joint problems or disease. For the duration of their sensitivity they are regarded as being suitable for needle or pressure treatment. These points may therefore be thought of as identical to the 'tender' points described by Lawrence Jones in his strain/counterstrain method, discussed later in this chapter (p. 58).

Alarm points, Associated points, Akabane points

There are, in traditional acupuncture, a number of key points which are most likely to become painful in relation to particular visceral dysfunction. These have been classified as Alarm points.

These are presented below, and the following general information may make their employment easier:

- The Alarm points are found only on the ventral surface of the body, each point being associated with one of the 12 meridians and its functions. Six of the points are on the midline, the others are bilateral. Tenderness elicited by palpation of an Alarm point may indicate dysfunction of the organ related to the point. In traditional acupuncture, if sensitivity is noted on light pressure, there is an associated energy deficiency. If heavy pressure is required, then the condition relates to an energy excess.
- Associated points lie on the back of the body, and these are all on the Bladder meridian, which runs parallel to the spine, bilaterally. Each Associated point is related to one of the meridians and its function. The same assumed relationship with energy deficit or excess exists, as in Alarm points (sensitivity on light pressure = deficiency, and on heavy pressure = excess). There are also a few extra Associated points, as illustrated (Fig. 4.3). Spontaneous pain at any of these listed points indicates a disorder in that meridian, and its associated organ or function.
- Akabane points are found on the fingers and toes, being the terminal points of the meridians. Sensitivity of any of these is said to relate to dysfunction and imbalance of energy in that meridian. Electronic measurement of these points (Melzack et al 1977) is performed in a number of modern electroacupuncture systems such as EAV. Manual testing is common, and was obviously the method used

before electrical methods arrived on the scene. These points are all bilateral.

Location of Alarm points

Alarm points (Table 4.1 and Fig. 4.2) are on the anterior surface of the body. Spontaneous pain at any point is considered to indicate a disorder of the affiliated meridian. If tenderness is elicited on light pressure a deficiency of energy in the meridian is assumed, whereas tenderness elicited on heavy pressure indicates an excess of energy in the meridian.

These are reflex points for meridian function and awareness of the roles apparently played by the various meridians in body energy economics is necessary to evaluate the significance of re-

actions which produce tenderness in Alarm points.

Table 4.1 Alarm points

			Acupuncture point
Point 1	Lung		LU1
Point 2	Liver		LV14
Point 3	Gall bladder	Bilateral	GB24
Point 4	Kidney		GB25
Point 5	Spleen		LV13
Point 6	Large intestine		ST25
Point 7	Heart constrictor		VC17
Point 8	Heart		VC14
Point 9	Stomach		VC12
Point 10	Triple heater		VC5
Point 11	Small intestine		VC4
Point 12	Bladder		VC3

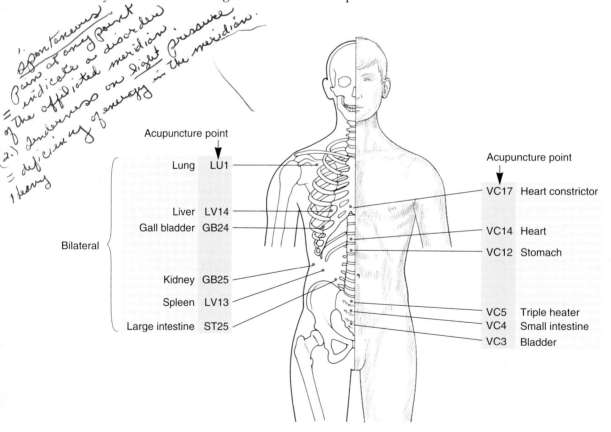

Figure 4.2 The location of Alarm points, which lie on the anterior surface of the body. If spontaneous pain develops in any alarm point, the associated meridian is thought to be involved. If light pressure produces tenderness, an 'energy deficiency' is considered to exist; if heavy pressure produces tenderness, an 'energy excess' is assumed. An understanding of the organs and functions associated with particular meridians is necessary in order to utilise these points therapeutically or diagnostically.

Location of Associated points

Associated points are on the dorsum of the body (Fig. 4.3). Spontaneous pain is thought to indicate a disorder in the meridian associated with it. Tenderness elicited on light pressure indicates a deficiency in energy in that meridian, and tenderness elicited on heavy pressure indicates an excess of energy in the associated meridian. These points are all on the Bladder meridian and their associations are given in Table 4.2. The points are slightly lateral to the median line bilaterally and are also reflex points for the meridians with which they are associated.

Location of Akabane points

Akabane points (Table 4.3 and Fig. 4.4) represent the terminal points of the meridians. Sensitivity of these is thought to relate to imbalance in the energy of the meridian. Comparative sensitivity shows relative imbalance in organ (energy) systems. Manual or electronic testing is possible.

Table 4.2   Associated points

Meridian		Bladder meridian point
Point 1	Lung	B13
Point 2	Heart constrictor	B14
Point 3	Heart	B15
Point 4	Governor vessel	B16
Point 5	Liver	B18
Point 6	Gall bladder	B19
Point 7	Spleen	B20
Point 8	Stomach	B21
Point 9	Triple heater	B22
Point 10	Kidney	B23
Point 11	'Sea of Energy'	B24 (Extra associated point)
Point 12	Large intestine	B25
Point 13	Small intestine	B27
Point 14	Bladder	B28

BENNETT'S NEUROVASCULAR REFLEX POINTS
(Martin 1977)

A wide degree of clinical experience resulted in an American chiropractor, Dr Terrence Bennett, reaching the conclusion that there was a group

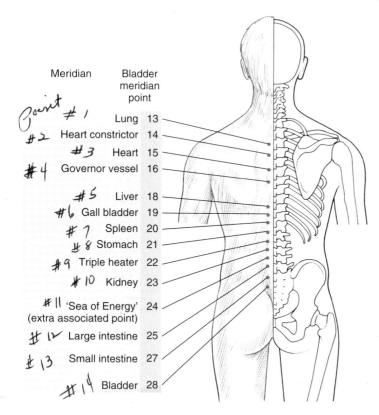

Meridian		Bladder meridian point
Lung	13
Heart constrictor	14
Heart	15
Governor vessel	16
Liver	18
Gall bladder	19
Spleen	20
Stomach	21
Triple heater	22
Kidney	23
'Sea of Energy' (extra associated point)	24
Large intestine	25
Small intestine	27
Bladder	28

Figure 4.3   Location of Associated points, which lie on the dorsal surface of the body slightly lateral to the median line bilaterally. If spontaneous pain develops in any associated point, the allied meridian is thought to be involved. If light pressure produces tenderness, an 'energy deficiency' is considered to exist; if heavy pressure produces tenderness, an 'energy excess' is assumed. An understanding of the organs and functions associated with particular meridians is necessary in order to utilise these points therapeutically or diagnostically.

Table 4.3 Akabane points

Points on Feet	Points on Hands
1. Spleen	7. Large intestine
2. Liver	8. Heart constrictor
3. Stomach	9. Triple heater
4. Gall bladder	10. Heart
5. Kidney	11. Small intestine
6. Bladder	12. Lung

of previously unknown reflexes available for diagnostic and therapeutic use, which he termed neurovascular reflexes. He described his work in a series of lecture notes, which were compiled and published by Ralph Martin, after Bennett's death, as *Dynamics of Correction of Abnormal Function* (Martin 1977). The major points are listed in Chapter 5, which deals with diagnostic procedures.

Bennett describes the tissues which are palpated as altered in texture, being contracted or indurated, in much the same way as Chapman's reflexes (see below, p. 53). His method of treatment calls for a slight degree of pressure, which he describes as 'only minimal, enough to render the tissues semi-anaemic, which is adequate stimulus'.

Experience indicates that the light pressure should be accompanied by slight stretching of the skin. In accordance with the views of Karel Lewit (1992), gentle stretching of the skin induces reflex activity when hyperalgesic (sensitised) skin zones are used therapeutically. When hyperalgesia occurs, skin becomes less elastic, with greater adherence to the underlying fascia and with lowered resistance to electricity.

In Bennett's system the skin is stretched with the minimum of force, so as to take up the slack, by the fingertips being drawn lightly apart. In most cases, if the area involves any degree of soft tissue dysfunction, a lack of anticipated elasticity will be noted in the skin as this distraction takes place. By maintaining the slight stretch on the tissues, a yielding occurs, and it is after this that a pulsation sensation should normally be felt. John Thie (1973) describes this pulsation sensation thus:

A few seconds after contact is made, a slight pulse can be felt, at a steady rate of 70 to 74 beats per minute. This pulse is not related to the heartbeat, but is believed to be the primitive pulsation of the microscopic capillary bed, in the skin.

Bennett insisted that the contact be maintained until a response was noted in the form of the tissue altering, relaxing and, most importantly,

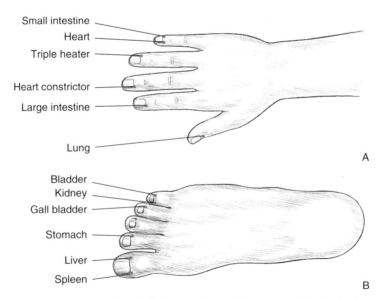

Small intestine
Heart
Triple heater
Heart constrictor
Large intestine
Lung

A

Bladder
Kidney
Gall bladder
Stomach
Liver
Spleen

B

Figure 4.4A,B Location of Akabane points, which represent the terminal points of the 12 meridians. Sensitivity of the points is thought to relate to imbalance in related organs (energy) systems. Both manual and electronic testing of these points is possible.

until the operator became aware of the presence of pulsation. This could arrive within a few seconds or take some minutes to emerge. The variable related directly to the patient and his condition. Bennett termed the pulsation felt as the 'arteriole pulse' because, he stated, 'It is the beginning of the system, at the junction of the artery and the arteriole, that controls the metabolism. The sensation of pulsation is essential,' he states. 'It has to be there, or else we are not accomplishing anything.' Together with this, the change in tissue feel is important. 'The tissues under your fingers begin to relax as you work for a few moments; you sense the degree of tension releasing. When it releases that is all you can do.'

Some points are purely diagnostic, others are used for treatment, and some are both. For example, the coronary reflex in the 2nd thoracic interspace on the left, which is a palpable area of tissue change and which is sensitive to the patient, is diagnostic only (not illustrated). Awareness of Bennett's reflex areas may be found to be a useful addition to the range of available therapeutic and diagnostic knowledge. In using neuromuscular technique, in its diagnostic mode, the tissues being evaluated will yield a multitude of sensitive points. Some of these may correlate with Bennett's findings, and they may then be used as part of an overall assessment as to the nature of the dysfunction affecting the patient. They may, of course, also be used, as Bennett intended, as a system in their own right, for assessing and treating visceral and functional physiological changes and pathology. A number of Bennett's points have been incorporated into the methods of applied kinesiology, notably the points on the cranium, which are used for treating emotional disturbances.

Among the cautions issued by Bennett are:

* Do not over treat the points on the cranium (2 to 3 minutes is a maximum)
* In hyperthyroid cases, do not treat the thyroid and pituitary reflexes at the same visit (one should be treated, and alternated with the other at a subsequent visit)
* If the heart is enlarged then the 3rd rib, at the midclavicular line, should not be treated
* Aortic sinus reflex should be treated before any of the brain reflexes are contacted

* If the ovary is being treated then the thyroid should receive prior attention.

A list of Bennett's reflex points will be found (p. 52) in Chapter 5, which deals with diagnostic applications of NMT.

CHAPMAN'S REFLEXES

(Mannino 1979, Owens 1980, Walther 1988) A 'neurolymphatic' reflex pattern, widely used in osteopathic and chiropractic methodology, was first described by Chapman and Owens. In an earlier work (Chaitow 1965) I discussed these reflexes as follows:

The reflexes of Chapman that I intend to discuss are not the whole picture – being only a part of the visible portion of the iceberg – but of immense value nonetheless. Drs Chapman and Owens first reported on Chapman's original findings in the late 1930s. A revised edition of their work has been published by the Academy of Applied Osteopathy.

The surface changes of a Chapman's reflex are palpable. They may best be described as contractions located in specific anatomical areas and always associated with the same viscera. In describing each organ reflex Chapman normally indicated tissue reflex areas, occurring anteriorly and posteriorly. These reflexes found in the deep fascia are described as 'gangliform' contractions. These contractions vary in size from a pellet to a large bean and are located anteriorly in the intercostal spaces near the sternum. Similar tissue changes are found in those reflexes occurring on the pelvis. The tissue changes found in reflexes located on the lower extremities are described as 'stringy masses' or 'amorphous shotty plaques'. Those reflexes occurring posteriorly along the spine, midway between the spinal processes and the tips of the transverse processes are of a more oedematous nature.

The value of the reflexes

Since the location of these palpable tissue changes is constant in relation to specific viscera it is possible to establish the location of pathology without knowing its nature. The value of these reflexes is threefold:

1. As diagnostic aids
2. They can be utilised to influence the motion of fluids, mostly lymph
3. Visceral function can be influenced through the nervous system.

The mechanism of the reflexes

As to the mechanism whereby these reflexes act, it would appear that, in so far as the intercostal reflexes are concerned, stimulation of the receptor organs which lie between the anterior and posterior layers of anterior intercostal fascia acts through the intercostal nerve, which enervates the external and internal intercostal muscles and thus, through the sympathetic fibres, affects the intercostal arteries, veins, lymph nodes, etc. Stimulation thus causes afferent and efferent vessels draining these tissues to increase or decrease, permitting lymph flow to be increased or decreased, thus affecting the drainage of the entire lymph system in the area. Through the sympathetic fibres associated with these tissues the lymph nodes of the vital organs are also affected.

Explaining results of neuromuscular technique

In my own mind I have no doubt that a knowledge of these reflexes goes a good way to explaining the sometimes startling results obtained through neuromuscular technique. Stanley Lief placed great emphasis on the intercostal spaces and the paravertebral areas – sites of many major neurolymphatic reflexes. He also stressed the importance of not over treating, a consideration which cannot be repeated too often.

Research evidence supports Chapman's reflex usefulness

In a trial conducted in order to assess the effects of forms of manipulation on blood pressure, one of the methods used was stimulation of a Chapman's reflex (Mannino 1979). A specific effect attributable to this treatment was noted. The point chosen for treatment was the one related to adrenal function. The trial involved treatment of this point, or a sham point, in which pressure was applied to either the real or a false point, for a total of 2 minutes, in a make or break circular motion. The point is located in the intertransverse space, on both sides of the 11th and 12th thoracic vertebrae, midway between the spinous processes and the tips of the transverse processes. The sham treatment involved the area between the 8th and 9th thoracic vertebrae (this point relates to small intestine problems, and would have no effect on the sort of condition being assessed in these trials).

The results showed no effect on blood pressure, but did indicate fascinating alteration in aldosterone levels. Many hypertensives are shown to have low renin/high aldosterone levels. This has an effect on the renal tubules, which causes retention of sodium. Abnormalities in aldosterone levels have been shown in populations with essential hypertension. There was a demonstrable and consistent fall in aldosterone levels within 36 hours of stimulation of the Chapman reflex for the adrenals, but no change at all in the levels when the sham points were stimulated. The delay in response suggested that the treatment had a tendency to interrupt, or damp down, a feedback to the adrenal medulla by the sympathetic nervous system. This could decrease the circulating amount of catecholamines, thereby diminishing their effect on the cardiovascular reflex which in turn exerts an influence on the renin–angiotensin–aldosterone axis. The question raised is why, if this effect is the result of the manipulation of a Chapman's reflex, was there no observed lowering of blood pressure? The researchers considered that this may have been the result of an inadequate time allowance for the development of a lowering effect. In the use of drugs which effect aldosterone levels, blood pressure is not lowered for between 5 and 7 days. Whether or not this suggestion is valid, the effect on aldosterone levels, via stimulation of the adrenal point, shows that these reflexes have a potent and predictable effect.

An element of disinformation has been forthcoming regarding the so-called neurolymphatic reflexes of Chapman, and it is important that this be corrected.

Raymond Nimmo and James Vannerson (1973) writing in the *Receptor* – the journal of the organisation which used (in the 1960s) to teach Nimmo's technique (receptor-tonus technique) a method of soft tissue manipulation with more than a passing similarity to aspects of NMT – stated:

Research has not borne out the presumption [by Chapman] of a neurolymphatic reflex. Muscle fibres, which alone have the specific function of constricting vessels, do not exist in the walls of lymph vessels, except for a few fibres in the thoracic duct, and a few large trunks. These are sparsely located, and have little effect in lymph fluid propulsion.

These two authors then deride Chapman's assertion that the reflexes could exist at specific sites, which they term 'fantastic.

The first part of their statement is in contradiction to Gray's *Anatomy* (Gray 1973, p. 715) which tells us that lymph moves in a number of ways. Filtration occurs, generated by filtration of fluid from the capillaries. There is also a degree of movement engendered by contraction of surrounding muscles, which compress lymph vessels, the movement of which is determined by the presence of valves. This muscular contraction is dependent upon normal activity, and muscular contraction–relaxation sequences. Lymph is further capable of being moved, in such regions, according to Gray, by massage movements. Pulsating arterial vessels, in close proximity, also assist lymph movement, as does respiratory movement. Finally, and in contradiction of Nimmo and Vannerson, Gray states: 'The smooth muscle in the walls of the lymphatic trunks is most marked just proximal to the valves; stimulation of sympathetic nerves accompanying the trunks, results in contraction of the vessels; the intrinsic muscle of the vessels thus probably aids the flow of the lymph.'

Since we may note that stimulation of cutaneous structures is capable of producing marked sympathetic responses, the possibility certainly exists that the term 'neurolymphatic reflex', as described by Chapman, may indeed be an accurate description of the phenomenon.

Beryl Arbuckle (1977) writes of Chapman's reflexes:

The diagnostic value of these reflexes is amazing. For instance, a female having severe pain in the right lower quadrant of the abdomen, presents several possibilities, but the offending organ may well be located by means of the reflexes, the positive one showing whether the disturbance is due to appendix, cecum, tube or ovary. With a degree of understanding of the interrelation of the endocrine glands, and of the importance of the lymphatics and the autonomic

distribution, the therapeutic value of these considerations can be shown clinically. There is a definite sequence which must be followed, in the management of these reflexes, to produce desired results, and, if not so applied, just as surely as the misapplication of any other therapy, further confusion of the body mechanism will result.

The second point made by Nimmo and Vannerson (relating to the specificity of the reflex sites) may be more valid, inasmuch as the factor of anatomical individuality is concerned. Points of the body surface are never likely to be precisely identifiable by description of anatomical position. However, a general identification as to site is possible. McBurney's point for example, if present in appendicitis, is usually located within a few degrees of its commonly described location. There are exceptions of course, and in the inscrutable manner of the Orient, the Chinese have taken this well into account, in describing the locations of acupuncture points. The invention of the 'human inch', which takes account of the individual anatomical proportions of each person, allows for such individualisation. In terms of the charts and maps to be found in this text, the same factor should be borne in mind. The positions are approximate, since variations will exist from person to person.

Dysfunction in soft tissues is, however, palpable, and not dependent upon maps. Thus the general guidelines provided by charts are useful, but cannot take the place of palpatory skills.

A complete illustrated list of Chapman's reflexes will be found in Chapter 5 (p. 75), which deals with diagnosis using NMT.

CONNECTIVE TISSUE MASSAGE

Another system which uses reflex effects diagnostically as well as therapeutically is connective tissue massage (CTM). CTM involves 'rolling' the tissues in order to achieve reflex and local effects. According to Ebner (1962) the palpable reflex tissue changes utilised in diagnosis and treatment in CTM methodology can take any of the following forms:

- Drawn-in bands of tissue
- Flattened areas of tissue

CMT =
Connective
Tissue
massage

- Elevated areas, giving the impression of localised swelling
- Muscle atrophy or hypertrophy
- Osseous deformity of the spinal column.

The strokes pull and stretch the tissues, and it is suggested that the method's effectiveness is based on a viscerocutaneous reflex. Bischof and Elmiger (1960) explain:

The specific mechanical stimulation of the pull on connective tissue seems to be the adequate stimulus to elicit the nervous reflex. Connective tissue massage acts first on the sympathetic terminal reticulum in the skin. The smallest branches of the autonomic nervous system contact the impulses activated by the pulling strokes to the sympathetic trunk and the spinal cord. The impulses travel from the skin either through a somatosensory spinal nerve via a posterior root ganglion to the grey matter or over the vascular plexus to the same segmental sympathetic ganglion or to the ganglion of the neighbouring segment, through the ramus communicans albus to the posterior root and grey matter of the spinal cord. They terminate either directly or by means of the internuncial neurons at the efferent autonomic root cells.

In the efferent pathway the impulses travel from the autonomic lateral horn, or the intermediolateral column, over the anterior root, ramus communicans albus, to the segmental sympathetic ganglion or to the ganglion of the neighbouring segment and finally to the diseased organ. The origin of the connective tissue reflex zones and the influence of the CTM depend on the relationship between the function of the internal organs, vessels, and nerves as well as the tissues of the locomotor apparatus, which descend from the same metamere.

Clara reminds us that the human embryo is composed of many homogeneous primitive segments (metameres) that are arranged serially. This arrangement is concerned with the meso-derm and the tissue regions derived from it – sclerotomes, myotomes, dermatomes, (ectoderm), angiotomes and nephrotomes. Secondly, the ectoderm participates in the segmentation (metamerism) since in each of the primitive segments or metameres one corresponding spinal nerve enters. The skin over the segment is also innervated, and in this way the segmentation is projected to the skin. This embryonal connection between the primitive segment and the spinal nerve (dermatome) develops early and remains unchanged postembryonically. Head was the first to point out that the internal organs that develop from the entoderm correspond to certain spinal cord segments, although the ento-derm does not participate in the segmentation. The relationship between tissues and their spinal root innervation is the scientific foundation for CTM and other forms of segmental therapy. Most investigators differ little in their reports concerning the segmental connections of the internal organs. Different schemes have been proposed by Hansen, Keegan, Dejerine and others to relate skin topography with the internal organs and reference to the cited texts on the subject (Bischof & Elmiger 1960, Ebner 1962) is suggested for further information.

During and after connective tissue massage, there are a number of reflex reactions including vasodilatation and diffuse or localised sweating. Some of these reflexes do not seem to be seg-mental in nature. For example, dilatation of the upper extremity blood vessels occurs when the pelvis is treated by CTM. The maximal skin temperature increase occurs about half an hour after CTM is discontinued and persists for an hour or so. It is of interest that the vasodilatory effect of CTM is as pronounced, or even more pronounced, after lumbar sympathectomy.

Some of the reactions to CTM are normal autonomic responses such as pleasant fatigue, bowel movements and diuresis. Oedema is markedly reduced and hormonal distribution is seen to achieve a degree of balance. Aspects of CTM are similar to NMT, and the 'skin rolling' methods used in some body areas are virtually identical in application. The effects are therefore interesting from a comparative point of view.

Research evidence into clinical effectiveness of CTM in cases of anxiety

A Scottish hospital undertook a trial in which a small group of patients attending a general psychiatric outpatient clinic were treated with connective tissue massage (JPR, 1983). The research was carried out at Bangour Village Hospital, near Broxburn in West Lothian.

The group selected presented with symptoms of impaired peripheral circulation, muscular tension, and pain. A frequent complaint was of sleep impairment, which was not associated with any particular pathology, and which was resistant to even large doses of hypnotic drugs. Those selected for the trial responded poorly to drugs, and were unable to learn standard relaxation techniques.

Connective tissue massage (CTM) was applied. An initial diagnostic assessment was made, using a specific massage stroke, applied systematically to the back. This was a form of subdermal traction, or deep stroking, which stimulates the autonomic branch of the nervous system. Patients reported a slight sensation of scratching or cutting. Where tissues were particularly tense when treated in this way, the sensation was stronger, being described as deep, dull pressure, or a sharp cutting sensation, both unrelated to the actual pressure being applied. A flare reaction of the tissues followed, and in some cases a weal developed. This sometimes persisted for some hours. The treatment proper consisted of a series of strokes which moved systematically through the back, each treatment lasting some 30 to 45 minutes, followed by a period of rest. Patients reported a feeling of warmth, and of being 'peaceful', and frequently fell asleep immediately. The night's sleep following treatment was reported generally to be deep and refreshing. The usual length of a course was 10 treatments, and these ceased either when patients reported the disappearance of symptoms, or when no further improvement was seen to be forthcoming. A positive response often involved profuse sweating during treatment, and this was sometimes unilateral.

A number of measurements and tests were conducted during the rest phase, after treatment. Arousal was tested by the playing, over a period, of 20 loud noises.

The physiological responses of the patients were recorded. Among the findings were that 4 out of 5 patients had a reduction in response to stress (randomly occurring loud noises) after CTM. This was of significant proportions. EMG activity, recorded on the frontalis muscle, showed that there was a significant decrease in response in 3 cases. Skin resistance was measured every minute during the rest period, and during the periods of stimulation with noise. EMG measurements were also recorded on the forearm extensor muscles. The findings

were that in 2 subjects there was a significant increase in skin resistance, indicating lowered arousal, and 2 other subjects showed reduction in forearm extensor EMG activity. The other patient showed inconclusive effects. All subjects showed a significant response in one or more of the psychophysiological parameters. After cessation of treatment, 3 out of 5 patients ceased use of drugs completely, and the other 2 required diazepam in only small doses. All reported diminution of symptoms. The researchers report that the differences noted in response, between EMG findings in the frontalis muscle and forearm extensor, is of interest, since the former is more reactive in depressive illness, and the latter is more so in cases of agitation.

It is significant that patients responded in their own way. There were no consistent findings, apart from overall reduction in evidence of symptoms and better sleep patterns. This supports the hypothesis that each individual has a unique pattern of response to stress, and that this pattern is consistent, regardless of the type of stress endured. The response to nonspecific therapy, such as CTM, allows the response of the individual to continue to be individual. They therefore utilise the beneficial aspects of the therapy in their own way, to meet the needs of their unique physiology.

The evidence resulting from this trial is that CTM is a useful tool in dealing with the consequences of psychiatric disturbances, anxiety and agitation. Clinical experience indicates that similar results may be derived from treatment utilising NMT. This is particularly relevant to problems involving sleep disturbance, such as is common in chronic fatigue syndrome and fibromyalgia – especially where anxiety forms one of the causal features (or results) of these widespread problems.

Electroacupuncture and trigger points

In their discussion of 'myodysneuria' (yet another name for fibrositis/fibromyalgia), Kleyhans and Aarons (1974) discuss the factors which initiate and which disperse trigger points. They believe that electroacupuncture owes much of its efficacy

Box 4.1 Possible symptoms from trigger points

Deep aching pain; headache; paraesthesia; menstrual pain; giddiness; weakness; shortness of breath; spasm; swallowing difficulty; blurred vision; sensitivity to light; tinnitus; anorexia; nausea; palpitation; oedema; excessively dry, oily or moist skin; depression; tension and poor concentration.

Table 4.4 Areas of inhibition and excitation with flexor and extensor responses in the knee

Motion of Knee	Area of Inhibition	Area of Excitation
Flexion	Over extensors only	Over rest of limb
Extension	Over flexors only	Over rest of limb

in such treatment to the fact that galvanic dispersement of trigger points occurs with its use. They maintain that most, if not all, trigger points can be dispersed by 'pressure techniques, ultrasound or galvanism, without recourse to the use of procaine injections or the use of chilling techniques'.

Having palpated and located the trigger point, and proved its ability to reproduce pain or other symptoms in a target area, stimulation of the point (i.e. pressure, stretching methods such as muscle energy technique etc.) can be carried out to deactivate it.

Among the symptoms which they list – and, of course, with which Travell and Simons are in agreement – as possibly deriving from trigger points are those given in Box 4.1.

Fuchs' system

M. Blashey (1961), dealing with limb rehabilitation, describes the research of Julius Fuchs, a German orthopaedist who died in 1953. Fuchs' system used supporting structures of a part elastic material and part non-elastic material, arranged so that antagonistic muscle groups were supported in such a way as to produce 'kinetic fields'. These fields were 'kinetically facilitating' where elastic tissue was used and 'kinetically impeding' where inelastic tissue was used. However, where sensory nerve damage had occurred in the skin overlying these muscles, no kinetic effect was obtained. It was found that only light pressure on the muscular structures involved was required to produce what Fuchs termed the 'orthokinetic' effect.

From this research we can learn a good deal about the reflex effect of light manipulation on the overlying tissue of affected muscles. Does there exist a specific function or structure or both,

connecting skin surface with underlying muscle, in a direct and specific manner? It seems so.

Hagbarth (1952) has shown that both flexor and extensor responses can be elicited in a definite structural pattern. In the knee, for example, the flexors can be stimulated from the skin of the entire limb apart from the skin overlying the extensors. (In his experiments he was using the cat as a model but later work has shown it to be valid for humans). The skin overlying the extensors is excitatory for the extensors. The converse applies, so that all skin covering the flexors is inhibitory for the extensors. This is summarised in Table 4.4. These effects were obtained thermally, electrically and by tactile stimulation which did not need to be heavy. The 'skin motor areas' or 'orthokinetic fields' do not correspond in distribution to the skin fields of cutaneous nerves or with segmental arrangements.

To summarise this finding: there is a definite functional connection between a muscle and the portion of skin that covers it. They are integrated so that muscle is excited by stimuli within its own skin area. This area will be inhibitory to the antagonist of the underlying muscle.

Jones' tender points (Fig. 4.5)
(Jones 1980)

In his evolution of the 'strain and counterstrain' functional manipulative approach to the normalisation of hypertonicity, Lawrence Jones described a series of 'points' which he had identified. These sensitive areas were, Jones discovered, related to specific strains and stresses in the musculoskeletal system, and were used by the therapist as monitors while the area was being guided into a position of ease, during which process there was both a reduction in sensitivity in the palpated tender point as well as a relaxation (increased ease) of the stressed tissues associated with it.

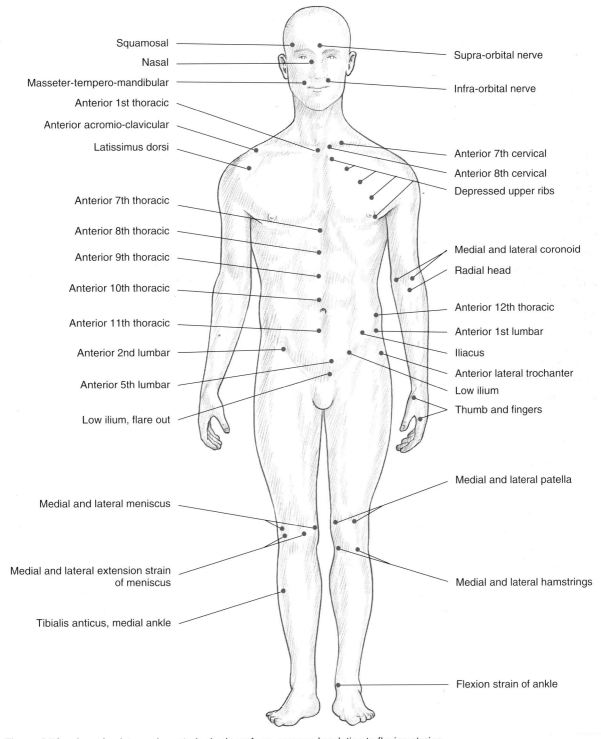

Squamosal

Nasal

Masseter-tempero-mandibular

Anterior 1st thoracic

Anterior acromio-clavicular

Latissimus dorsi

Anterior 7th thoracic

Anterior 8th thoracic

Anterior 9th thoracic

Anterior 10th thoracic

Anterior 11th thoracic

Anterior 2nd lumbar

Anterior 5th lumbar

Low ilium, flare out

Medial and lateral meniscus

Medial and lateral extension strain
of meniscus

Tibialis anticus, medial ankle

Supra-orbital nerve

Infra-orbital nerve

Anterior 7th cervical

Anterior 8th cervical

Depressed upper ribs

Medial and lateral coronoid

Radial head

Anterior 12th thoracic

Anterior 1st lumbar

Iliacus

Anterior lateral trochanter

Low ilium

Thumb and fingers

Medial and lateral patella

Medial and lateral hamstrings

Flexion strain of ankle

Figure 4.5A   Jones' points on the anterior body surface, commonly relating to flexion strains.

Figure 4.5   Location of Jones' tender points, which are bilateral in response to specific strain (acute or chronic) but are shown on only one side of the body in these illustrations. The point locations are approximate and will vary within the indicated area, depending upon the specific mechanics and tissues associated with the particular trauma or strain.

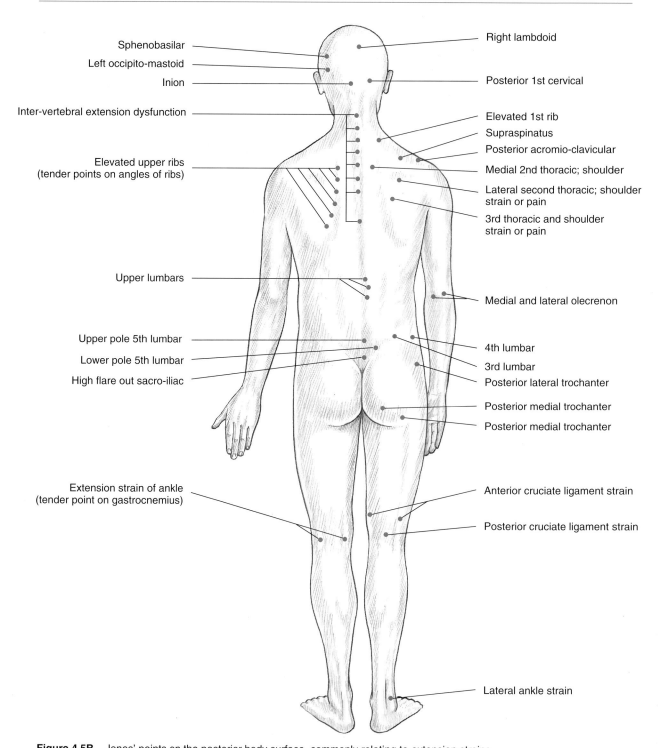

Figure 4.5B Jones' points on the posterior body surface, commonly relating to extension strains.

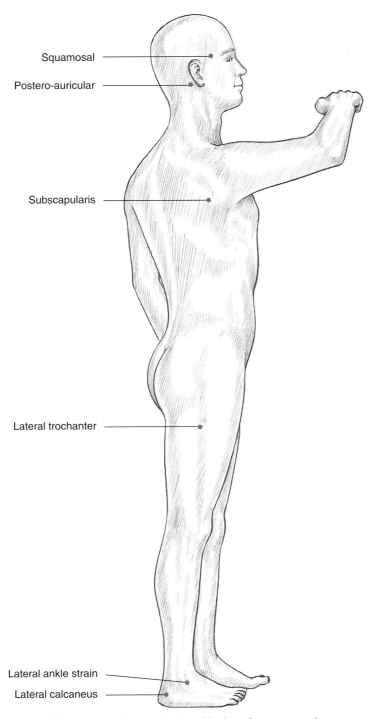

Squamosal

Postero-auricular

Subscapularis

Lateral trochanter

Lateral ankle strain

Lateral calcaneus

Figure 4.5C   Jones' points on the lateral body surface, commonly relating to strains involving sidebending or rotation.

In many ways these points, sensitive to palpation but not usually areas in which the patient was previously aware of pain, are similar to Ah Shi points in traditional Chinese medicine – spontaneously tender points (Chaitow 1991).

Significantly perhaps, as the area being treated is positioned in 'ease' so that tenderness vanishes from the tender point, a degree of ischaemic compression/inhibitory pressure/acupressure would be taking place. It is worth considering that the benefits noted in terms of pain relief and reduction in contraction or spasm, could relate in some part to the resulting inhibitory/endorphin release action as well as to the subsequent improvement in circulation through the tissues and neurological modulation produced by the placing of the tissues into a situation of 'ease'.

Periosteal pain points (PPP)
(Adapted from Lewit 1992)

These painful areas (see Table 4.5) usually relate to acute or chronic contraction of associated muscles and tendons.

Felix Mann, pioneer acupuncture researcher and author, describes periosteal acupuncture as being more effective than ordinary acupuncture in a number of conditions. He lists the sites given in Table 4.6 amongst the common sites usefully employed in this approach. Clinical experience indicates that NMT ischaemic compression techniques and muscle energy methods are as likely as traditional needling to produce benefit when treating these points.

Confusion?

The soft tissues are of major importance to the body's economy, structural integrity and well being. They are also a major source of pain and dysfunction and, as must now be obvious, of reflex disturbances.

The various theories, methods and descriptive terminologies relating to the many point systems and classifications of 'points' are significant inasmuch as neuromuscular technique offers the opportunity for accessing and using their potential. If we accept that there are many ways of

Table 4.5 Periosteal pain points

Site	Muscular/joint implication
Pain on head of metatarsals	Dropped arch, flat foot
Spur on calcaneum (pain on pressure)	Tight plantar aponeurosis
Pain on tubercle of tibia	Tight long adductor/possible hip dysfunction
Pain on head of fibula	Biceps femoris tightness
Posterior superior iliac spine tenderness	Various possible implications, involving low back, gluteal and sacroiliac region
Lateral aspects of symphysis pubis	Adductors tight. Hip or sacroiliac dysfunction
Pain on coccyx	Gluteus maximus tightness, possibly piriformis or levator ani involvement
Crest of ilium – pain	Tight quadratus lumborum/gluteus medius and/or lumbodorsal dysfunction
Pain on greater trochanter	Tight abductors/hip dysfunction
Pain on lumbar spinous processes (especially L5)	Tight paraspinal muscles
Pain mid-dorsal spinous processes	Lower cervical dysfunction
Pain spinous process of C2	Levator scapular tight: C1–2, 2–3, dysfunction
Pain on xyphoid process	Rectus abdominus tight. 6–8 rib dysfunction
Pain on ribs, on mammary or axillary line	Pectoralis tightness. Visceral dysfunction referred to here
Pain at sternocostal junction upper ribs	Scalenus tightness
Pain on claviclemedial aspect	Tight sternocleidomastoid
Pain transverse process of atlas	Tight sternocleidomastoid and/or recti capitis lateral Atlanto–occipital dysfunction
Pain on occiput	Upper cervical or atlas dysfunction
Pain on styloid process of radius	Elbow dysfunction
Pain on epicondyles	Local muscular or elbow dysfunction
Pain at deltoid attachment	Scapulohumeral dysfunction
Mandibular condyles painful	TMJ dysfunction. Tight masticators

(Adapted from Lewit 1992)

Table 4.6 Periosteal acupuncture points and associations

Site	Associated with
1. Appropriate transverse cervical process	Headache, migraine, inter-scapular pain and cervical spondylosis
2. Area of sacroiliac joint	Low back pain, sciatica without neurological deficit, testicular pain
3. Coracoid process	Painful shoulder joint
4. Medial condyle tibia	Knee pain, without advanced pathology
5. Neck of femur	Hip pain, without major changes evident on X-ray
6. Lateral aspect of posterior spine of lower lumbar vertebrae	If sacroiliac joint (2 above) does not yield benefit, these areas may be used

looking at and interpreting the same phenomenon then it will be an easy step to acknowledging that an acupuncture point and a trigger point and a Chapman's reflex point (for example) can all be the self-same point – but with different aspects of its reflex potential being considered in each classification.

Neuromuscular technique can (with other modalities) be used as an effective measure to detect and eliminate noxious trigger points and areas which generate or help to maintain dysfunction or which influence reflexive activity. Such dysfunction can take the form of muscular weakness, muscular contraction, pain, vasodilatation, vasoconstriction, tissue degeneration, gastrointestinal disturbances, sympathetic nervous system abreactions, respiratory and a myriad other disorders including emotional and 'psychological' disorders such as anxiety.

Noxious (pain producing) points which are the end result of various forms of stress imposed on the tissues housing them may reside in either hypertonic or hypotonic muscle, or in ligamentous or fascial tissues, or in apparently normal tissues. When active, such points will always be sensitive to correctly applied pressure and can often be neutralised by manual pressure or a combination of chilling and manual pressure and stretching.

In the treatment sections there will be discussion as to methods for locating and treating such points.

REFERENCES

Arbuckle B 1977 The selected writings of Beryl Arbuckle. National Osteopathic Institute and Cerebral Palsy Foundation

Baldry P 1993 Acupuncture, trigger points and musculoskeletal pain. Churchill Livingstone, Edinburgh

Bischof I, Elmiger G 1960 Connective tissue massage. In: Licht E (ed) Massage, Manipulation and Traction. New Haven, Connecticut

Blashy M 1961 Manipulation of the neuromuscular unit via the periphery of the CNS. Southern Medical Journal August

Bosey J 1984 Acupuncture and Electro-Therapeutics Research 9(2): 79–106

Botek S 1985 Acupuncture and Electro-Therapeutics Research 10(3): 241

Chaitow L 1965 An introduction to Chapman's reflexes. British Journal of Naturopathy (Spring)

Chaitow L 1991 Acupuncture treatment of pain. Healing Arts Press, Vermont

DiGiovanna E 1991 An osteopathic approach to diagnosis and treatment. Lippincott, Philadelphia

Ebner M 1962 Connective tissue massage. Churchill Livingstone

Ernst M 1983 Acupuncture and Electro-Therapeutics Research 8(3/4): 343

Gray H 1973 Gray's anatomy, 35th edn. Longman

Hagbarth K 1952 Excitatory inhibitory skin areas for flexor and extensor motoneurons. Acta Physiologica Scandinavia

Jones L 1980 Strain and counterstrain. Academy of Applied Osteopathy, Boulder

JPR 1983 Anxiety states: preliminary report on the value of connective tissue massage. Journal of Psychosomatic Research 127(2): 125–129

Kleyhans, Aarons 1974 Myodysneuria and acupuncture. Digest of Chiropractic Economics

Lewit K 1992 Manipulative therapy in rehabilitation of the locomotor system. Butterworths

Lewith G, Kenyon J 1984 Social Science and Medicine 19(12): 1367–1376

Mann F 1983 International Conference of Acupuncture and Chronic Pain. September 1983

Mannino J 1979 The application of neurological reflexes to the treatment of hypertension. Journal of the American Osteopathic Association 79(4): 225–230

Martin R (ed) 1977 Dynamics of correction of abnormal function. Ralph Martin, Sierra Madre

Melzack R, Stillwell D, Fox E 1977 Trigger points and acupuncture points of pain. Pain 3: 3–23

Nimmo R, Vannerson J 1971 Receptor tonus technique. The Receptor 12(1): 47

Northup G 1941 The role of the reflexes in manipulative

therapy. Journal of the American Osteopathic Association 40: 521–524

Owens C 1980 An endocrine interpretation of Chapman's reflexes. American Academy of Osteopathy

Serizawe K 1976 Tsubo: vital points for oriental therapy. Japan Publications, San Francisco

Takeshige C 1985 Acupuncture and Electro-Therapeutics Research 10(3): 195–203

Thie J 1973 Touch for health. DeVorss, California

Travell J, Simons D 1992 Myofascial pain and dysfunction, vol. 2. Williams and Wilkins, Baltimore

Wall P, Melzack R 1989 Textbook of pain. Churchill Livingstone, Edinburgh

Walther D 1988 Applied kinesiology. SDC Sysems, Pueblo

5

Diagnostic methods

In previous chapters we have dipped into the vast amount of information that exists relating to the neuromuscular component of the human framework. A great number of diagnostic aids

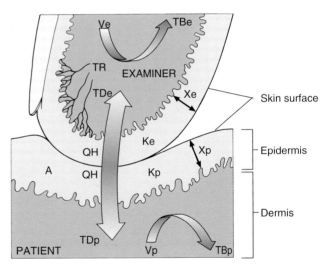

Figure 5.1   This diagram depicts some of the physical and physiologic factors that affect the thermoreceptor (TR) discharge rate and consequently the temperature sensed in an examiner's skin in contact with a patient's skin. The temperature and its rate of change of the examiner's thermoreceptors are functions of the net effects of the time that the tissues are in contact, their contact area (A), the temperatures (TBe and TBp) and volume flow rates (Ve and Vp) of blood perfusing the examiner's and patient's skin, epidermal thickness (Xe and Xp) and thermal conductivity (Ke and Kp) of both, dermal temperature (TDe and TDp) of both, as well as of the net heat exchange rate (QH) between the two tissues. QH is strongly affected by the heat transfer properties of material trapped between the two skin surfaces, for example, air, water, oil, grease, hand lotion, dirt, tissue debris and fabric (Adams, Steinmetz, Heisey, Holmes and Greenman 1982).

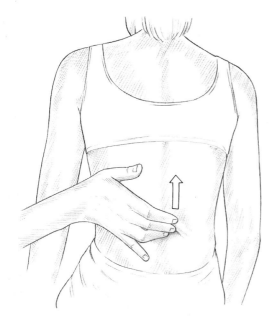

Figure 5.2 Light 'skin on skin' palpation can give indications of deeper dysfunction due to modification of sympathetic and circulatory activity.

exist for discovering just what is happening when aspects of this network of tissues malfunction. The great beauty of neuromuscular technique, as devised by Lief, is the way in which diagnostic and therapeutic movements are combined. The thumb, as it glides close to the spinal attachments of the paraspinal musculature, is assessing the tissue tone, density, temperature etc., and at the same moment is capable of treating those tissues that indicate dysfunction. The response of the searching thumb or finger to whatever information the tissues impart, can be immediate. The use of greater or lesser degrees of pressure, varying in direction and duration, allows the practitioner to judge and treat at the same time and with great accuracy (Figs 5.1 and 5.2).

If treatment of musculoskeletal dysfunction is to be focused and meaningful, a diagnostic or assessment plan is required. Whilst local muscular changes will become more apparent as treatment progresses, an overall diagnostic picture is required to enable a coherent plan to emerge and for prognosis and progress to be judged.

NEUROMUSCULAR TECHNIQUE – ASSESSMENT/DIAGNOSIS

If therapeutic intervention is to be structured and organised and something other than hit and miss there is a basic need for evaluation and assessment of the way the mechanical component of the body is adapting to its current situation, of the extent of changes from the norm and of the ways in which patterns of pain, malco-ordination and restriction are interacting. These changes might involve reflexively active structures such as myofascial trigger points, locally traumatised areas, fibrotic alterations, shortened and/or weakened muscles, joint restrictions and/or general/systemic factors (such as exist in arthritic conditions).

NMT provides a diagnostic/assessment tool and also offers, when it switches from its assessment to its actively therapeutic mode, a means whereby very precisely focused and modulated degrees of force can be directed towards influencing restricted tissues. Myofascial release techniques, as well as ischaemic compression (osteopathic inhibitory technique), can be applied to precise targets via the contacting thumb or finger in NMT. Perhaps NMT's greatest usefulness in assessment relates to the opportunity it offers for the identification of local soft tissue dysfunction in a gentle, non-invasive manner. In the USA as well as in the UK, the focus of many therapists utilising NMT in recent years has been towards the identification and treatment of myofascial trigger points (and the often widespread musculoskeletal dysfunction which produces or is associated with them).

PALPATION

There is no valid substitute for skilful palpatory diagnosis in ascertaining the relatively minute structural changes – primary or reflex – that often have far-reaching effects on the body's economy.

It is generally agreed that the pads of the figures are the most sensitive portion of the hand available for use in diagnosis. Indeed, the combination of the thumb and first two fingers is the finest mechanism, and can be adapted to conform with the variable areas under palpatory consideration.

Palpatory diagnosis
(Baldry 1993, Beal 1983, DiGiovanna 1991, Travell & Simons 1983, 1992)

One of the most successful methods of palpatory diagnosis is to run the pads of a finger or several fingers extremely lightly over the area being checked, assessing changes in the skin and thereby the tissues below it. After localising any changes in this way, deeper periaxial structures can be evaluated by means of the application of greater pressure. There are a number of specific changes to be sought in light palpatory examination. This applies to both acute and chronic dysfunction. Among these are:

1. *Skin changes*. (Lewit 1992) Over an area of acute or chronic dysfunction, skin will feel tense and will be relatively difficult to move or glide over the underlying structures.

The skin overlying reflexively active areas such as trigger points (or active acupuncture points) tends to produce a sensation of 'drag' as it is lightly stroked – due to increased hydrosis. There is also an apparent undulation sensation, a rising and falling, palpable on a light stroke – described illustratively as 'hills and valleys'.

The skin will lose its fully elastic quality, so that on light stretching (taking an area of skin to its easy resistance barrier on stretching) it will test as less elastic than neighbouring skin.

The skin above reflexively active structures will also be more adherent to the underlying fascia, something which will be evident in any attempt to glide it or roll it, when compared with normal areas.

All of these changes can become apparent in the application of neuromuscular palpation/assessment strokes.

2. *Induration*. A slight increase in diagnostic pressure will ascertain whether or not the superficial musculature has an increased indurated feeling. When chronic dysfunction exists the superficial musculature will demonstrate a tension and immobility indicating fibrotic changes within

and below these structures. These changes will be further discussed in the text dealing with the application of basic spinal and abdominal NMT (Chs 6 and 7).

3. *Temperature changes*. In acute dysfunction a localised increase in temperature may be evident. In chronic lesion conditions there may, because of relative ischaemia, be a reduced temperature of the tissues. This usually indicates that fibrotic alterations have occurred.

4. *Tenderness*. Tenderness of palpated tissues requires investigation. Is the tissue inflamed? Is the local area reflexively active? What is the nature and cause of the sensitivity?

5. *Oedema*. An impression of swelling, fullness and congestion can often be obtained in the overlying tissues in acute dysfunction. In chronic dysfunction this is usually absent having been replaced by fibrotic changes.

The questions which need to be asked when palpation elicits the sort of changes briefly covered above include:

- What am I feeling?
- What significance does it have in relation to the patient's condition/symptoms?
- How does this relate to any other areas of dysfunction I have noted?
- Is this a local problem or part of a larger pattern of dysfunction?
- What does this mean?

In deep palpation, the pressure of the palpating fingers or thumb needs to increase sufficiently to make contact with deeper structures such as the periaxial (paravertebral) musculature without provoking a defensive response. Amongst the changes which might be noted may be immobility, tenderness, oedema, deep muscle tension, fibrotic and interosseous changes. Apart from the fibrotic changes, which are indicative of chronic dysfunctions, all these changes can be found in either acute or chronic problems.

As Peter Lief (1963), son of the innovator of neuromuscular technique, explains:

Palpation is the main method of detection. Gross lesions are easily palpable but sometimes they are so minute that their detection presents considerable difficulty, especially to the beginner. It sometimes takes many months of practice to develop the necessary sense of touch, which must be firm, yet at the same time sufficiently light, in order to discern the minute tissue changes which constitute the palpable neuromuscular lesion.

The presence of a lesion is always revealed by an area of hypersensitivity to pressure, an area which may be better described as being a painful spot. After these have been detected and noted, specific attention is given to them in the subsequent treatments.

Brian Youngs (1964) has described what it is that the palpating fingers are seeking and finding and, since in NMT diagnosis and treatment often take place together, what they are achieving:

The changes which are palpable in muscles and soft tissues associated with reflex effects have been listed by Stanley Lief. They are essentially 'congestion'. This ambiguous word can be interpreted as a past hypertrophic fibrosis. Reflex cordant contraction of the muscle reduces the blood flow through the muscular tissue and in such relatively anoxic regions of low pH and low hormonal concentration, fibroblasts proliferate and increased fibrous tissue is formed. This results in an increase in the thickness of the existing connective tissue partitions – the epimysia and perimysia and also this condition probably infiltrates deeper between the muscle fibres to affect the normal endomysia. Thickening of the fascia and subdermal connective tissue will also occur if these structures are similarly affected by a reduced blood flow. Fat may be deposited, particularly in endomorphic types, but fibrosis is most pronounced in those with a strong mesomorphic component – a useful pointer for both prognosis and prophylaxis.

Fibrosis seems to occur automatically in areas of reduced blood flow, e.g., in a sprained ankle – where swelling is marked and prolonged, in the lower extremities where oedema of any origin has been constant over a period, in the gluteals where prolonged sitting is a postural factor, and in the neck and upper dorsal region where psychosomatic tension is frequent to a marked degree – depending upon the constitutional background. Where tension is the aetiological factor, fibrosis seems teleological.

Many devices have been developed to ease the strain on muscles which tend to be permanently contracted, e.g., locking of the kneejoint, or the exact balance of the head on the shoulders, where only gentle contraction is needed to maintain postural integrity. If postural integrity is lost through some cause or another then the strain on the muscle may be eased by structural alteration and the increase of

fibrous tissue in the muscles acts to maintain normal position of the head. Fibrous tissue can then take the strain instead of the muscle fibres. It is this long-term homeostatic reflex which apparently operates in all cases of undue muscle contraction, whether due to strain or tension.

From this one can amplify Stanley Lief's beneficial effects of neuromuscular treatment as follows:

1. To restore muscular balance and tone.
2. To restore normal trophicity in muscular and connective tissues by altering the histological picture from a patho-histological to a physiologic-histological pattern with normal vascular and hormonal response.
3. To affect reflexly the related organs and viscera and to tonify them naturally.
4. To improve drainage of blood and lymph through the areas subject to gravitational or postural stasis, e.g., abdominal vessels not necessarily connected with viscera.
5. To reduce fatty deposits.

Thus the hyperaemia resulting from treatment automatically operates to reverse the original patho-histological picture and consequently normality will be approached.

In clinical terms it is safe to say that a chronic state of dysfunction exists if soft tissues have been consistently stressed for more than a few weeks, for after such a short period fibrotic adaptations begin to be palpable.

There is clinical evidence that trigger points have a consistent distribution and their localisation can be predicted by studying the patterns of referred dysfunction and pain to which they give rise. Similarly patterns of referred pain are predictable if the trigger point can be located (Travell 1957).

A patient with unexplained pain, the examination of which reveals no local cause, may well have trigger points feeding pain messages into the target area. Thus the point at which the patient feels pain and the point at which the pain originates are often not the same and knowledge of the reference patterns as illustrated in Chapter 3 is therefore desirable.

Whether treatment of trigger points consists of anaesthetic injections, acupuncture, cryotherapy or pressure and stretch techniques (NMT) the diagnostic aspect remains the same. Deep palpation and pressure on the located point must reproduce the symptoms in the target area in order to 'prove' the connection.

Other palpable changes

As well as trigger points there exist a number of palpable and often visible zones of soft tissue alteration involving reflex activity, including viscerosomatic activity in which diseased or stressed organs negatively influence soft tissues paraspinally and elsewhere (Bischof et al 1960) (Fig. 5.3). Some of these zones overlap and incorporate 'trigger' points and a general awareness and knowledge of their existence is useful if an understanding of what can being achieved in NMT treatment is to be more complete.

Since organs mainly receive their autonomic supply homolaterally, changes of a reflex nature will normally be found on the same side of the body surface. On the right side will be found the connective tissue reflex zones from the liver, gall bladder, duodenum, appendix, ascending colon

and ilium etc. On the left side will be found the reflex zones from the heart, stomach, pancreas, spleen, jejunum, transverse colon, descending colon and rectum etc. Central zones occur as a result of dysfunction in the bladder, uterus and the head. Changes on the homolateral side of the body occur due to dysfunction of the lungs, super renal glands, ovaries, kidneys, blood vessels and nerves on that side. According to Teiriche-Leube and Ebner (quoted in: Teiriche-Laube 1960) these changes in the connective tissue and muscles can take the following forms:

- Drawn in bands of tissues
- Flattened areas of tissue
- Elevated areas, giving the impression of localised swelling
- Muscle atrophy or hypertrophy
- Osseous deformity of the spinal column.

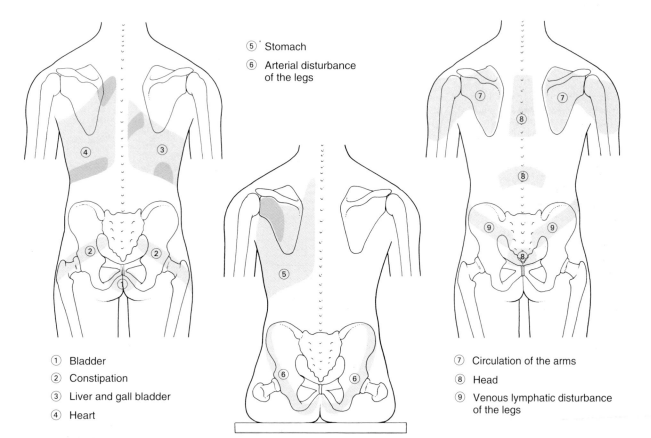

⑤ Stomach
⑥ Arterial disturbance of the legs

① Bladder
② Constipation
③ Liver and gall bladder
④ Heart

⑦ Circulation of the arms
⑧ Head
⑨ Venous lymphatic disturbance of the legs

Figure 5.3 Connective tissue reflex zones (after Ebner).

For Teiriche-Leube and Ebner's description of some of these zones see Box 5.1.

Using neuromuscular technique in its assessment mode as described in later chapters (Chs 6 & 7), or specialised skin diagnosis (see below, p. 72–75) these and other areas of soft tissue dysfunction can be readily located, identified and treated even if no obvious symptoms of the associated conditions or diseases are present. It is clear that tissue changes often precede the appearance of symptoms of underlying pathology and in this alone the diagnostic value of these zones is evident. Practitioners using German connective tissue massage claim that it is often possible to beneficially influence symptoms of organ dysfunction and to improve the function of these organs (liver, stomach etc.) by treatment of the congested fibrotic reflex zone. This is not, however, to be considered an end itself since it is clear that underlying causative factors and pathology (nutrition, infection etc.) must also be dealt with. However, the value of the neuromuscular tool should not be minimised.

Assessing dominant eye

In making a visual diagnosis it is important for the operator to be sure of the information he is acquiring. American osteopathic physician Edward Stiles (1984) makes a valuable contribution to this area by pointing out that it is often for reasons of position, in observing structure, that a student or practitioner fails to see what is obvious:

By being so positioned as to bring into play the non-dominant eye this becomes far more likely. The orientation of the subject in the field of view is determined by the position of the dominant eye, and thus it is essential to initially ascertain which eye this is.

Hold your hands straight out in front of you.

Box 5.1 Altered connective tissue zones resulting from disturbed organs and functions

1. **Bladder**.
   Small, 'drawn in' area above anal cleft. Iliotibial tract may be drawn in. Swelling lateral aspect of ankles.
   Symptoms – Bladder dysfunction. Cold feet and legs (below the knee).
   Rheumatic diagnosis.
2. **Constipation**.
   'Drawn in' band 2 to 3 inches (5–8 cm) wide running from middle third of the sacrum downwards and laterally.
   Symptoms – Tendency to, or actual constipation.
3. **Liver and gall bladder**.
   Large 'drawn in' zone over right thoracic region and a band along lateral costal border on the right side. Small 'drawn in' area between lower vertebral border of scapula to spine at the 5th and 6th dorsal level. 7th cervical area appears swollen or congested.
   Symptoms – Liver and gall bladder dysfunction and anyone who has suffered from hepatitis.
4. **Heart**.
   Tension over left thoracic region including lower costal margin. If hepatic circulation is involved right costal margin will also be affected. The area between the left scapula and 2nd and 3rd dorsal vertebrae will be indurated. Posterior aspect of axilla appears thickened.
   Symptoms – Coronary and valvular diseases of the heart.

5. **Stomach**.
   (a) Overlapping the heart zones (above).
   Symptoms – Stomach dysfunction.
   (b) Localised tension area below lateral aspect of the left scapular spine.
   Symptoms – Gastric ulcer and gastritis.
6. **Arterial disease of legs**.
   A V-shaped configuration of the buttocks when sitting is noticed rather than the normal rounded shape.
   Symptoms – Circulatory disturbance accompanied by angiospasm.
7. **Arms**.
   'Drawn in' areas over scapula extending over posterior deltoid.
   Symptoms – Circulatory arm and hand problems. Neuritis paraesthesia.
8. **Head**.
   (a) Thoracic area between scapulae.
   Symptoms – Insomnia and all types of headache.
   (b) Lower third of sacrum just above bladder zone.
   Symptoms – Headaches related to digestive dysfunction.
   (c) Just below origin of trapezius.
   Symptoms – Headaches due to tension.
9. **Venous lymphatic disturbance of the legs**.
   A tight band from middle third of sacrum, parallel to iliac crest laterally and anteriorly over gluteus medius.
   Symptoms – Cramp. Swollen legs in summer, varicose veins and paraesthesia.

Palms facing each other. Bring them together to make an aperture (gap) about one to two inches across. Looking through this aperture focus on an object across the room from you. Close first one eye and then the other. When the non-dominant eye is closed the image you see through the aperture will not change. When you close the dominant eye the image shifts out of the field of vision. The dominant eye is not always on the same side as the dominant hand. If dominant hands and eyes are on different sides, this can lead to problems of accurately assessing palpatory findings, and the advice given is to palpate with eyes closed, where possible, in such cases.

When assessing visually, make sure that the dominant eye is lined up with the area or object being viewed. In an example where assessment of the chest is being made, Stiles suggests that since most accurate visual information will be gained when the dominant eye is over the midline, the observation of the supine patient should be from the head of the table, and this should be approached from the side which brings the dominant eye closer to the patient.

Mackenzie's abdominal reflex areas

Youngs (1964) points out that Sir James Mackenzie established a clear relationship between the abdominal wall and the internal abdominal organs (Mackenzie 1909). Mackenzie showed that organs which cannot react directly to painful stimuli (i.e. the majority) react by producing spasm and paraesthesia in the reflexly related muscle wall (the myotome) often augmented by hyperaesthesia of the overlying skin (dermatome).

The reflexes involved occur via the autonomic nervous system and can be viscerosomatic or, as has been shown by many researchers, including Lief, the origin can be somatic and the reflex therefore somaticovisceral.

Mackenzie's abdominal reflex areas are as illustrated (Fig. 5.4) and although there is sometimes a degree of individualisation it is

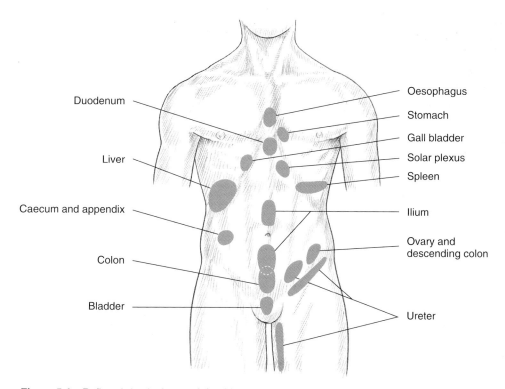

Figure 5.4 Reflex abdominal areas (after Mackenzie).

reasonable to state that the presence in abdominal muscles and connective tissues of contracted or sensitive areas indicates (in the absence of recent trauma or strain) some underlying dysfunction which is causing or resulting from the soft tissue lesion.

SKIN: REFLEX EFFECTS AND HYPERALGESIC SKIN ZONES (HSZ)

We have seen in the work of Mackenzie early in the 20th century, as well as later in the development and research into connective tissue zones evolving out of Bindegewebsmassage in Germany, that the surface of the body provides evidence of internal derangement, and that it is possible to influence the interior by application of reflexively powerful stimuli from the surface.

Kiyomi Koizumi, of the State University of New York Department of Physiology, has studied the relationship between the skin surface and the internal structures of the body (Koizumi 1978) and in this research using animals it was found that stimulation of the skin of the abdomen produced profound inhibition of intestinal movement. Stimulation of the skin produces an increase in sympathetic fibre activity innervating the intestine, thereby inhibiting the mobility of the region. He notes that this is a strong effect, and that the intestine often became completely quiescent.

Stimulation of other skin areas, notably the neck, chest, fore and hindlimbs, inhibited sympathetic activity, and therefore actually augmented intestinal motility. Vagal involvement in these changes was thought to be minimal, for when the vagi were sectioned the same responses were still noted. Reflexes disappeared, however, when the sympathetic nerve supply to the intestine, the splanchnic nerves, were sectioned. The somatic sympathetic reflex from the abdominal skin is a spinal reflex, whereas the reflexes originating from the other skin areas were thought to be a supraspinal reflex. The researcher points out that, whereas the parasympathetic system plays little part in these reflexes, its involvement increases aspects of emotional reactions. If we consider the involvement of these mechanisms

in affecting internal function, via stimulus applied to the skin, we may better appreciate the findings of Chapman (Owen 1963), Bennett (Arbuckle 1977) and others, in their work on the multitude of reflex areas, which they have so painstakingly charted, and which are available to us.

The sometimes dramatic effects obtained by the use of connective tissue massage methods can also be seen to relate to the patterns of therapeutic and diagnostic opportunities, which this knowledge opens.

For example, various techniques are available to us in diagnosing from, and treating, the cutaneous structures for reflex effect. These include skin rolling as well as the delicate 'skin distraction' or stretching method, advocated by Lewit (1992). He discusses hyperalgesic skin zones which, if we reflect, are likely to be present in the skin overlying most, if not all, areas of reflex activity. Lewit points out a major advantage which awareness of hyperalgesic skin zones (HSZ) offers. This is that, unlike the eliciting and mapping of areas, points or zones, which rely upon the subjective reporting of the patient, these areas are palpable to the operator. A popular method of noting relative tension in skin is to 'roll' it. A fold of skin is formed, and this is rolled between the fingers (see Fig. 8.10). This method may produce some discomfort, or even transient pain, but is useful in that the increased tension and visibly thicker skin fold thus produced (as compared with surrounding tissues) is diagnostic of a HSZ.

Lifting skin folds (diagnostic)

The methods used in connective tissue massage are designed to obtain a picture of the mobility of the various layers of the connective tissue, as well as an idea of their consistency. One such method involves the lifting of skin folds, with the patient sitting. The skin is gripped between thumb and fingers, with care being taken not to pinch the fold (Fig. 5.5). The fold comprises sufficient tissue to allow it to be lifted away from the fascial layer. This is usually performed, starting at the lower costal margin, and going up as far as the region of the shoulders. In some

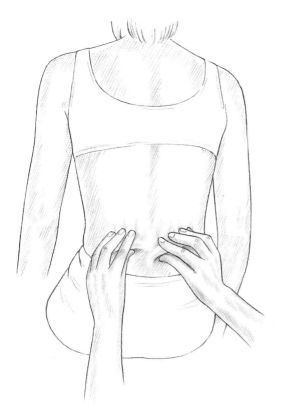

Figure 5.5 Skin folds can be lifted from the underlying fascial layer to test for restrictions which may indicate local or reflexive dysfunction.

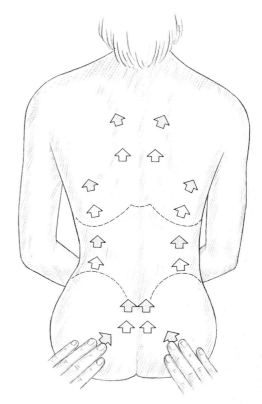

Figure 5.6 Testing and comparing skin and fascial mobility as bilateral areas are 'pushed' to their elastic barriers.

areas, especially overlying the mid-dorsal region, if there is any dysfunction involving the liver, gall bladder, stomach or heart, restriction of tissue elasticity will be noted. By lifting two folds simultaneously, right and left, it is possible to compare the relative freedom of these tissues.

Stretching superficial tissue (diagnostic)

A second method may be used, in which relatively smaller areas are assessed with patient prone or seated. With fingers lightly flexed, and using only enough pressure to produce adherence between the fingertips and the skin, a series of short pushing motions is made simultaneously with both hands, which stretches the tissues (Fig. 5.6). Usually the pattern of testing goes from inferior to superior, sometimes in an obliquely

diagonal direction. The patient is seated, and the operator works from behind, testing tissues from the buttocks to the shoulders.

Areas investigated, direction of stretch of tissues, and implications of reduced elasticity include:

1. The buttocks; stretching tissue from the ischial region, towards the lateral borders of the sacrum (arterial and constipation zone).
2. From the posterior aspect of the trochanters, towards the iliac crests (venous lymphatic and arterial disturbances of legs).
3. From the trochanters, towards sacroiliac joints (venous lymphatic zone).
4. Over the sacrum, working from the apex towards the upper sacral segments (bladder and headache zones).
5. Over the lumbar region, on either side of the spine, working upwards (kidney zone).
6. Bilaterally up the spine, from lower costal region to the mid-thoracic level (liver and gall

bladder zone (right side), and heart, stomach (left) and pulmonary dysfunction (on either side)).

7. Between the scapulae (headache zone).

8. Over the scapulae, from inferior angle, towards spine of scapula (arm zone).

Normal variations will exist independent of reflex activity and in individuals carrying increased adipose tissue, there will be a generally greater degree of tension or adherence noted, as compared to a thinner individual. An older person's skin will feel looser, in comparison to a younger individual's. The skin over the lumbar region is naturally less mobile than other regions.

Note that it is adherence ('tightness of tissues to each other') which is being assessed, and this may or may not be accompanied by sensitivity. In connective tissue massage an assessment of this sort is made regularly, as it is both diagnostic and prognostic, showing the rate of progress or lack of it, and providing a unique insight into visceral and functional status.

Skin distraction (diagnostic and therapeutic)

Lewit describes a 'new' method, which he finds reliable, painless and therapeutically very useful. Any area of skin may be thus assessed, large or small, with fingertip or hand contact.

In a small area, the fingertips (both index fingers) or index and middle finger tips of both hands, are placed close together, resting on the tissues to be tested. By separating the fingers the skin is stretched (Fig. 5.7). A minimum of force is used, in order to simply take out the slack in the skin. The 'easy' end-position is noted, as is the degree of 'springing' in the tissues. This is compared in several directions, over the area, and comparison is also made with the presumably healthy tissue, on the contralateral side. If a HSZ is present, then a greater degree of resistance will be noted, after the slack has been taken up. Where there is such resistance, if the end-position of stretch is held for approximately 10 seconds, the resistance will be felt to ease, and the normal physiological degree of springing will then be noted. This is measurable, and by marking the first stretch position with a skin pencil, and marking the stretch position available after 'release of the tissue', a measurable improvement will usually be noted.

The techniques may be used even for small areas (e.g. between the toes). These may be stretched by fingertip (light) pressure and separation. Larger areas are contacted by the ulnar border of the hands. The hands are crossed and placed on the tissue to be tested. Separation of the hands introduces stretch to take up the slack.

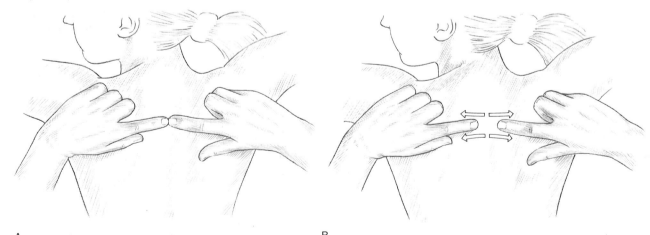

A   B

Figure 5.7A,B Hyperalgesic skin zones which lie above reflexive dysfunction (e.g. trigger points) are identified by means of the sequential stretching to their elastic barrier of local areas of skin. A series of such stretches indicates precisely those areas where elasticity is reduced as compared with surrounding tissues. These are then tested for sensitivity and potential to cause referred pain by the application of ischaemic compression (inhibition).

Having introduced this initial degree of stretch, resistance (end-feel) is then noted. If the tissues are resistant to stretch, and springiness is absent, the maintenance of the stretch (painless) achieves a release of the tissues.

All trigger points, tender points, connective tissue zones, Mackenzie's abdominal areas etc., are characterised by the presence of HSZ in the overlying tissues. This very useful tool allows easy identification of reflex activity and is itself an ideal form of treatment of these reflexes, and further provides accurate evidence of the subsequent situation. Techniques for treating skin and superficial tissue are further discussed in later chapters (Chs 6 & 7).

Scar tissue often results in the presence of HSZ's around the scar and these frequently become focal points of reflex activity. Acupuncture is a useful method of treating any very sensitive aspect of the scars themselves (Baldrey 1993).

CHAPMAN'S REFLEXES IN DIAGNOSIS AND TREATMENT

The reflexes described by Chapman are now commonly termed 'neurolymphatic' reflexes. These can be used in diagnosis and treatment and as a guide to the effectiveness of treatment. In 1965 I described the technique for using these as follows (Chaitow 1965):

Treatment applied through these reflexes, as advocated by Chapman and Owens, consists of a firm but gentle rotary pressure imparted by the index or middle finger. The finger should not be allowed to slip. As these areas are acutely sensitive great care should be taken not to overtreat as the reflex will become fatigued and no benefit will be derived.

My current view coincides with the above method except that I now use a variable thumb pressure which fits in with the general neuromuscular technique. Knowledge of the exact location of the reflexes is of primary importance.

By gentle palpation the operator should first ascertain the presence of involved reflexes. The anterior reflexes should be tested first. If found to be present, the anterior reflex should be treated first, then the posterior counterpart of the involved anterior reflexes should be treated. The anterior reflex has, therefore, a dual role: namely, for diagnosis and then to initiate the reflex treatment. The anterior reflex is later of value to ascertain the effectiveness of treatment (after both anterior and posterior reflexes have been treated).

If, on repalpating the reflexes, there is no change in the feel or tenderness, the treatment should be repeated. If there is again no change it indicates either that the pathology is too great for rapid change, or that pathology is irreversible. It may also indicate that some musculoskeletal factor is maintaining the reflex. Primary treatment should then be directed at this factor rather than the reflex. The degree of treatment should be ascertained by palpation. Chapman and Owens described dosage of treatment in terms of seconds, but in practice I feel that anyone experienced in neuromuscular treatment would have the degree of sensory awareness required to 'feel' when sufficient treatment has been given.

I would stress that I have found the reflexes of Chapman useful in differential diagnosis and in the treatment of various conditions from spastic constipation to migraine – but always as a part of a broad approach to the patient as a whole. That they can influence lymphatic drainage dramatically, I have no doubt – I am less sure of the effect on visceral conditions but have found that the reflexes themselves provide an excellent guide to progress. If they are no longer present, then invariably the condition is progressing well.

Technique and charts for use of Chapman's reflexes (Fig. 5.8)

Chapman (Owen 1963) suggested a vibratory treatment in stimulating the neurolymphatic reflexes, lasting 10 to 15 seconds. He used fingertip pressure to impart the required energy, although thumb pressure of varying intensity is just as effective. This can be applied as a gradually intensifying pressure building up over 5 to 8 seconds, easing for 2 or 3 seconds and then repeated. Altogether this should not take more than half a minute. These points can be overtreated and the optimum time would seem to be from 15 to 30 seconds with the pressure (or

Table 5.1 Location of Chapman's neurolymphatic reflexes

No. symptoms/area	Anterior	Fig.	Posterior	Fig.
1. Conjunctivitis and retinitis	Upper humerus	5.8A	Occipital area	5.8C
2. Nasal problems	Anterior aspect of first rib close to sternum	5.8A	Posterior the angle of the jaw on the tip of the transverse process of the first cervical vertebra	5.8C
3. Arms (circulation)	Muscular attachments pectoralis minor to third, fourth and fifth ribs	5.8A	Superior angle of scapula and superior third of the medial margin of the scapula	5.8C
4. Tonsillitis	Between first and second ribs close to sternum	5.8A	Midway between spinous process and tip of transverse process of first cervical vertebra	5.8E
5. Thyroid	Second intercostal space close to sternum	5.8A	Midway between spinous process and tip of transverse process of second thoracic vertebra	5.8C
6. Bronchitis	Second intercostal space close to sternum	5.8A	Midway between spinous process and tip of transverse process of second thoracic vertebra	5.8E
7. Oesophagus	As No. 6	5.8A	As No. 6	5.8E
8. Myocarditis	As No. 6	5.8A	Between the second and third thoracic transverse processes. Midway between the spinous process and the tip of the transverse process	5.8D
9. Upper Lung	Third intercostal space close to the sternum	5.8A	As No. 8	5.8D
10. Neuritis of upper limb	As No. 9	5.8A	Between the third and fourth transverse processes, midway between the spinous process and the tip of the transverse process	5.8D
11. Lower Lung	Fourth intercostal space, close to sternum	5.8A	Between fourth and fifth transverse processes. Midway between the spinous process and the tip of the transverse process	5.8D
12. Small intestines	Eighth, ninth and tenth intercostal spaces close to cartilage	5.8A	Eighth, ninth and tenth thoracic intertransverse spaces	5.8C
13. Gastric hypercongestion	Sixth intercostal space to the left of the sternum	5.8A	Sixth thoracic intertransverse space, left side	5.8C
14. Gastric hyperacidity	Fifth intercostal space to the left of the sternum	5.8A	Fifth thoracic intertransverse space, left side	5.8F
15. Cystitis	Around the umbilicus and on the pubic symphysis close to the midline	5.8A	Upper edge of the transverse processes of the second lumbar vertebra	5.8F
16. Kidneys	Slightly superior to and lateral to the umbilicus	5.8A	In the intertransverse space between the twelfth thoracic and the first lumbar vertebra	5.8F
17. Atonic constipation	Between the anterior superior spine of the ilium and the trochanter	5.8A	Eleventh costal vertebral junction	5.8C
18. Abdominal tension	Superior border of the tension pubic bone	5.8A	Tip of the transverse process of the second lumbar vertebra	5.8D
19. Urethra	Inner edge of pubic ramus near superior aspect of symphysis	5.8A	Superior aspect of transverse process of second lumbar vertebra	5.8F
20. Depuytrens contracture, and arm and shoulder pain	None		Anterior aspect of lateral margin of scapulae, inferior to the head of humerus	5.8F
21. Cerebral congestion (related to paralysis or paresis)	(On the posterior aspect of the body) Lateral from the spines of the third, fourth and fifth cervical vertebrae	5.8A	Between the transverse processes of the first and second cervical vertebrae	5.8E

Table 5.1 (Cont)

No. symptoms/area	Anterior	Fig.	Posterior	Fig.
22. Clitoral irritation and vaginismus	Upper medial aspect of the thigh	5.8A	Lateral to the junction of the sacrum and the coccyx	5.8D
23. Prostate	Lateral aspect of the thigh from the trochanter to just above the knee. Also lateral to symphysis pubis as in uterine conditions (see No. 43)	5.8A	Between the posterior superior spine of the ilium and the spinous process of the fifth lumbar vertebra	5.8D
24. Spastic constipation or colitis	Within an area of an inch or two wide extending from the trochanter to within an inch of the patella	5.8A	From the transverse processes of the second, third and fourth lumbar vertebrae to the crest of the ilium	5.8C
25. Leucorrhoea	Lower medial aspect of thigh, slightly posteriorly (on the posterior aspect of the body)	5.8A & 5.8C	Between the posterior/superior spine of the ilium and the spinous process of the fifth lumbar vertebra	5.8D
26. Sciatic neuritis	Anterior and posterior to the tibiofibula junction	5.8A	1. On the sacroiliac synchondrosis 2. Between the ischial tuberosity and the acetabulum 3. Lateral and posterior aspects of the thigh	5.8C
27. Torpid liver (nausea, fullness malaise)	Fifth intercostal space, from the mid-mammillary line to the sternum	5.8B	Fifth thoracic intertransverse space on the right side	5.8C
28. Cerebellar congestion (memory and concentration lapses)	Tip of coracoid process of scapula	5.8B	Just inferior to the base of the skull on the first cervical vertebra	5.8E
29. Otitis media	Upper edge of clavicle where it crosses the first rib	5.8B	Superior aspect of first cervical transverse process (tip)	5.8C
30. Pharyngitis	Anterior aspect of the first rib close to the sternum	5.8B	Midway between the spinous process and the tip of the transverse process of the second cervical vertebra	5.8E
31. Laryngitis	Upper surface of the second rib, 2 or 3 inches (5–8 cm) from the sternum	5.8B	Midway between the spinous process and the tip of the second cervical vertebra	5.8E
32. Sinusitis	Lateral to the sternum on the superior edge of the second rib in the first intercostal space	5.8B	As No. 31	5.8E
33. Pyloric stenosis	On the sternum	5.8B	Tenth costovertebral junction on the right side	5.8F
34. Neurasthenia (chronic fatigue)	All the muscular attachments of pectoralis major on the humerus clavicle, sternum, ribs (especially fourth rib)	5.8B	Below the superior medial edge of the scapula on the face of the fourth rib	5.8D
35. Wry Neck (Torticollis)	Medial aspect of upper edge of the humerus	5.8B	Transverse processes of the third, fourth, sixth and seventh cervical vertebrae	5.8E
36. Splenitis	Seventh intercostal space close to the cartilaginous junction, on the left	5.8B	Seventh intertransverse space on the left	5.8C
37. Adrenals (allergies, exhaustion)	Superior and lateral to umbilicus	5.8B	In the intertransverse space between the eleventh and twelfth thoracic vertebrae	5.8F
38. Mesoappendix	Superior aspect of the twelfth rib, close to the tip, on right	5.8B	Lateral aspect of the eleventh intercostal space on the right	5.8C
39. Pancreas	Seventh intercostal space on the right, close to the cartilage	5.8B	Seventh thoracic intertransverse space on the right	5.8F

Table 5.1 (Cont)

No. symptoms/area	Anterior	Fig.	Posterior	Fig.
40. Liver and gall bladder congestion	Sixth intercostal space, from the mid-mammillary line to the sternum (right side)	5.8A	Sixth thoracic intertransverse space, right side	5.8F
41. Salpingitis or vesiculitis	Midway between the acetabulum and the sciatic notch (this is on the posterior aspect of the body)	5.8F	Between the posterior, superior spine of the ilium and the spinous process of the fifth lumbar vertebra	5.8D
42. Ovaries	The round ligaments from the superior border of the pubic bone, inferiorly	5.8B	Between the ninth and tenth intertransverse space and the tenth and eleventh intertransverse space	5.8D
43. Uterus	Anterior aspect of the junction of the ramus of the pubis and the ischium	5.8B	Between the posterior superior spine of the ilium and the fifth lumbar spinous process	5.8D
44. Uterine fibroma	Lateral to the symphysis, extending diagonally inferiorly	5.8B	Between the tip of the transverse process of the fifth lumbar vertebra and the crest of the ilium	5.8C
45. Rectum	Just inferior to the lesser trochanter	5.8B	On the sacrum close to the ilium at the lower end of the iliosacral synchondrosis	5.8F
46. Broad ligament (uterine involvement usual)	Lateral aspect of the thigh from the trochanter to just above the knee	5.8B	Between the posterior, superior spine of the ilium and the fifth lumbar spinous process	5.8D
47. Groin glands (circulation and drainage of legs and pelvic organs)	Lower quarter of the sartorius muscle and its attachment to the tibia	5.8B	On the sacrum close to the ilium at the lower end of iliosacral synchondrosis	5.8F
48. Haemorrhoids	Just superior to the ischial tuberosity. (These areas are on the posterior surface of the body)	5.8D	On the sacrum close to the ilium, at the lower end of the iliosacral synchondrosis	5.8D
49. Tongue	Anterior aspect of second rib at the cartilaginous junction with the sternum	5.8A	Midway between the spinous process and the tip of the transverse process of the second cervical vertebra	5.8E

squeeze) of a variable nature. If the patient is able to report a referred pain resulting from the pressure then pressure/treatment can be continued for up to a minute, with fluctuations in the degree of pressure, until the patient indicates a diminution in the referred pain or until the time has elapsed.

It is important to realise that the objective 'feel' of these contractions is unlikely to change during such treatment. Any changes resulting from the treatment will occur later, when homeostatic forces have come into operation. The variation in pressure during the treatment is more desirable than a constantly held degree of pressure, which may irritate and exacerbate the condition. In the Foreword to Owen's book *An Endocrine Interpretation of Chapman's Reflexes*, in which Owen describes his and Chapman's

research, noted osteopathic researcher Fred Mitchell recommends that pressure be applied by the pad of the middle finger. This should be maintained as a light direct pressure in an effort to decongest the fluid content of the palpable reflex point. Mitchell believes that the determining factor for the amount of treatment is whether a decrease in oedema takes place, or whether there occurs a dissolution of the gangliform contraction, together with reduction in the sensitivity of the point over a period of between 20 and 120 seconds. The stimulation threshold is being raised in these points and inhibition of noxious impulses is being achieved. There is nothing to be gained from achieving local pressure anaesthesia (numbing) by exaggerated effort. Reflexes that are not painful should not be treated – only an active (and therefore sensitive) reflex point requires attention.

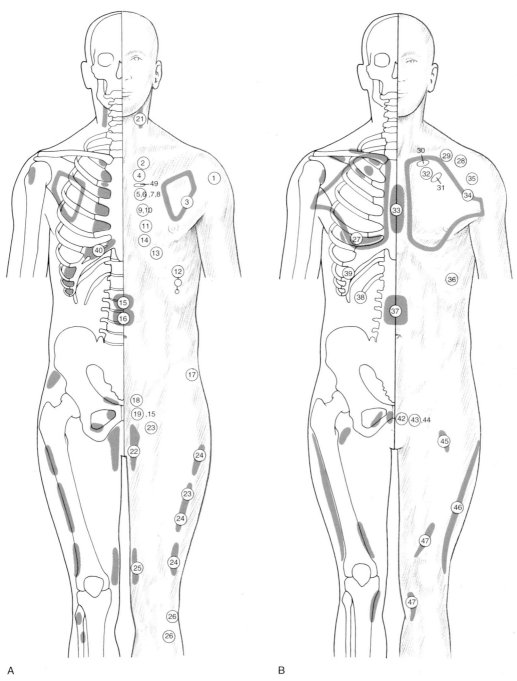

A B

Figure 5.8A,B Chapman's neurolymphatic reflex areas. Symptom/area numbers are as Table 5.1.

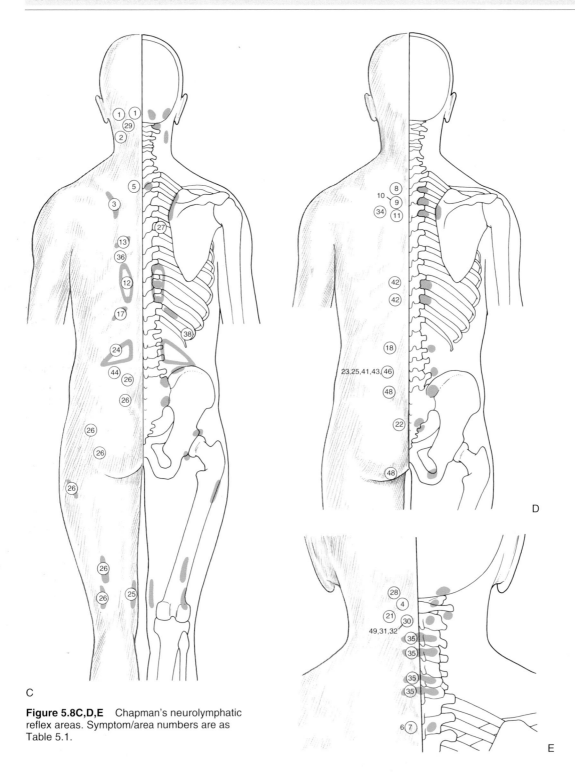

C

D

E

Figure 5.8C,D,E Chapman's neurolymphatic reflex areas. Symptom/area numbers are as Table 5.1.

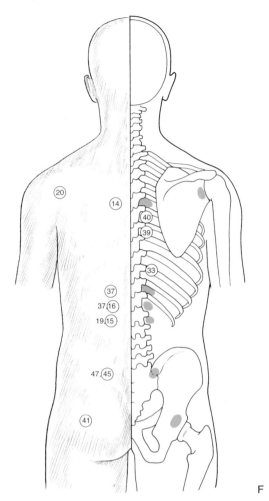

F

Figure 5.8F Chapman's neurolymphatic reflex areas. Symptom/area numbers are as Table 5.1.

The reflexes may be treated as part of a general neuromuscular treatment or on their own in accordance with the recommendations of Chapman, Owen and Mitchell, which suggest the treating of the reflexes by light digital pressure of the anterior reflex followed by the corresponding posterior reflex. The anterior point should then be re-examined and if there has been a palpable change, or if sensitivity has diminished, then no more action would be required. If no such change is found then the treatment to the anterior and then the posterior points is again carried out and if still no change is noted then it is assumed that pathology is too great for a rapid change or is irreversible or that there is a musculoskeletal factor maintaining the dysfunction.

If this approach is adopted then the grouping of reflexes into systems is a useful method. If one of a group is found to be active then all others in the group should be examined and, if active, treated; for example, the endocrine group comprises: prostate, gonads, broad ligaments, uterus, thyroid and adrenals. The gastrointestinal group comprises the colon, thyroid, pancreas, duodenum, small intestine and liver. The infections group comprises liver, spleen and the adrenals. The advice therefore is to use reflexes intelligently, treating only what is palpable and sensitive.

Some of the anterior reflexes (the ones which should, in theory, be treated first) lie on the posterior aspect of the body. These include those for haemorrhoids (No. 48) cerebellar congestion (No. 21) leucorrhoea (No. 25) and salpingitis (No. 41).

It is suggested that reference be made to the above-mentioned book (Owen 1963) for more detailed study. Table 5.1 gives the reflex by name, number and description of location together with an indication of which drawing illustrates it (it was not possible to incorporate all the drawings onto one picture without creating a confusing series of overlaps). It is suggested that the practitioner learns to search appropriate areas for the type of sensitive tissue changes which represent the superficial manifestation of these reflexes and to use the drawings and the list in Table 5.1 to become familiar with the patterns and groups of these important aids to healing. The illustrations will aid the practitioner in locating these useful diagnostic and therapeutic areas.

BENNETT'S NEUROVASCULAR REFLEXES (Note these will be sensitive to light pressure if active.) (See Figs 5.9A,B,C and Box 5.2.)

Aetiology

Speransky (1943) has stated that the nervous system contains a record of the past history of the organism. For the practitioner, the signs present in the musculoskeletal system constitute a map of past and present dysfunctions. It presents him

Box 5.2 Bennett's neurovascular reflexes

Reflex name	Site

Reflex name — **Site**

1. **Parotid gland** — Raised area on masseter when jaw clenched
Diagnostic and treatment point. Associated conditions: Prostate problems, mumps, premenstrual problem, mastitis, lymphatic stasis.

2. **Cardiac sphincter** — Tip of xyphoid process
Diagnostic and treatment point. If sensitive may relate to incompetent sphincter, heartburn.

3. **Liver** — Midclavicular line; right 5th intercostal
Diagnostic and treatment point.

4. **Gall bladder** — Below costal cartilages right 9, 10, 11th ribs
Diagnostic and treatment point. All points mentioned are treatment points; only 11th rib point is diagnostic. Pain may be noted as far lateral as mid-axillary line.

5. **Pancreas** — Medial to 6th and 7th rib heads. 1 inch below xyphoid process
Diagnostic point. 5th and 6th costal cartilages right and left.

6. **Pyloris** — Lower border of umbilicus
Diagnostic and treatment point.

7. **2nd segment of duodenum** — 1 inch and 45° above umbilicus on right
Diagnostic and treatment point.
Note: Order of treatment in this region should follow sequence of pyloris–duodenum–pancreas–liver–gall bladder.

8. **3rd portion of duodenum** — 1 inch and 45° above umbilicus on left
Diagnostic and treatment point.

9. **4th portion of duodenum** — 1 inch and 45° lateral and below umbilicus (left)
Diagnostic and treatment point.

10. **Kidneys** — Tip of 8th rib. Bilateral
Diagnostic and treatment point.

11. **Iliocecal valve** — On right side midway between anterior–superior iliac spine and umbilicus
Diagnostic and treatment point.

12. **Internal rectal sphincter** — On left midway between anterior/superior iliac spine and umbilicus
Diagnostic and treatment point.

13. **Appendix** — Directly over the organ
Diagnostic and treatment point.

14. **Bladder** — Just above pubic arch on midline
Diagnostic and treatment point.

15. **Prostate/uterus** — Symphysis pubis
Diagnostic and treatment point.

16. **Spermatic cord/ovary** — Approx. $1-1\frac{1}{2}$ inches either side of bladder reflex (note thyroid to be treated when ovaries receiving attention)
Diagnostic and treatment point.

17. **Super-renal** — One finger width below tip 12th rib. Diagnostic point is tip of 12th rib.
Diagnostic and treatment point.

18. **Anterior pituitary** — Right, lateral aspect of eyebrow
Diagnostic and treatment point.

19. **Posterior pituitary** — Left, lateral aspect of eyebrow
Diagnostic and treatment point.

20. **Thyroid** — Over the organ
Diagnostic and treatment point.

21. **Carotid sinus** — On carotid artery, below angle of jaw
Diagnostic and treatment point.

22. **Aortic sinus** — Manubriosternal junction on ridge, or just inferior
Diagnostic and treatment point.

23. **Heart tone** — Sternal end of 3rd rib. Contact on cartilage (left)
Diagnostic and treatment point.

24. **Sub-clavian lymphatics** — Just inferior to and slightly medial to midpoint of clavicle
Diagnostic and treatment point.

25. **Femoral lymphatics** — On Poupart's ligament. Midway between symphysis pubis and anterior superior iliac spine
Diagnostic and treatment point.

26. **Maxillary sinus** — Lateral to nares; bilaterally
Diagnostic and treatment point.

Box 5.2 (Cont)

Reflex name	Site
27. **Bronchial region**	Midway between manubrium sternum and episternal notch *Diagnostic and treatment point.*
28. **Frontal-emotional**	Frontal eminences of forehead *Diagnostic and treatment point.*
29. **Vagal**	2 inches superior and 2 inches posterior to external auditory meatus *Diagnostic and treatment point.*
30. **Parietal**	2 inches superior and 3 inches posterior to external auditory meatus *Diagnostic and treatment point.*
31. **Temporal-emotional**	Midway between outer aspect of eye and external auditory meatus. Just superior to zygomatic bone *Diagnostic and treatment point.*
32. **Anterior fontanelle**	Over anatomical area *Diagnostic and treatment point.*
33. **Midsylvian**	1 inch superior to anterior aspect of external auditory meatus *Diagnostic and treatment point.*
34. **Fissure of Rolando**	Approx $1\frac{1}{2}$ inches posterior to anterior fontanelle *Diagnostic and treatment point.*
35. **Frontal eye fields**	$1\frac{1}{2}$ inches superior to frontal eminences *Diagnostic and treatment point.*
36. **Extrinsic eye muscles**	Superior to eyelids with closed eyes *Diagnostic and treatment point.*
37. **Posterior fontanelle**	Over anatomical area *Diagnostic and treatment point.*
38. **Menopause-glandular**	$\frac{1}{2}$ inch inferior and lateral to posterior fontanelle *Diagnostic and treatment point.*

All the points on the cranium are useful for treating emotional and stress conditions. Those marked 'emotional' are the strongest. Light pressure only is suggested. Reference to these reflexes will be found in the chapter on treatment techniques (Ch. 6).

---

with the opportunity to treat, alleviate and prevent further dysfunction.

Apart from palpation for tissue changes and reflex trigger areas, diagnosis should involve an evaluation of the gross stress patterns and postural factors. Each patient is an individual challenge, and indeed this challenge is renewed at each visit. Thus, whilst the mechanics of treatment are similar, the emphasis will probably be different at each visit. It is important that the patient understands this, and the nature of the problem as well as the goal desired. A cooperative patient will accept the time and effort required to achieve that goal. Observation of the dynamic posture or body in motion gives an idea of balance, posture, gravitational stress, gross structural anomalies etc. Observation of certain body areas in individual movement will then help the understanding of their stress patterns, restrictions etc. The practitioner must learn to appreciate the arrangement of the various body structures and their inter-relationships. The myofascial tensions can then be visualised. When these gross and local postural patterns in active and passive modes have been observed an overall impression can be added to the palpatory impressions, both superficial and deep, which the hands can evaluate with the patient standing, supine or prone. By lightly passing the hands over the various structures, alterations in tissue density and configuration can be felt. The deeper palpation to localise the dysfunction can then be performed or left to the neuromuscular treatment where diagnosis coincides with treatment.

A history will have been taken prior to observation, palpation, and mobility tests and such history should be comprehensive, taking note of traumatic incidents, habits, occupational positions and postures, emotional state and history, congenital deformity, surgery as well as general medical history and specific details of the presenting problems.

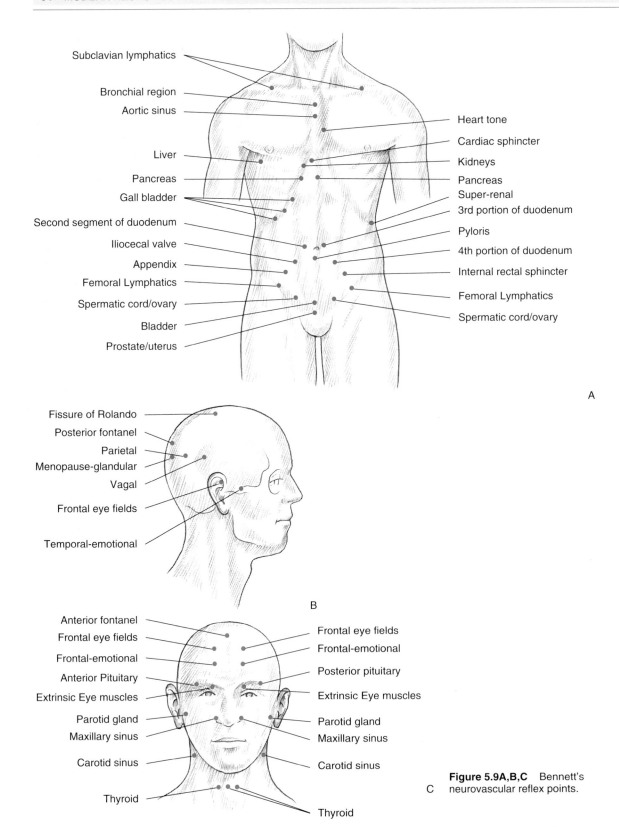

Subclavian lymphatics

Bronchial region

Aortic sinus

Liver

Pancreas

Gall bladder

Second segment of duodenum

Iliocecal valve

Appendix

Femoral Lymphatics

Spermatic cord/ovary

Bladder

Prostate/uterus

Heart tone

Cardiac sphincter

Kidneys

Pancreas

Super-renal

3rd portion of duodenum

Pyloris

4th portion of duodenum

Internal rectal sphincter

Femoral Lymphatics

Spermatic cord/ovary

A

Fissure of Rolando

Posterior fontanel

Parietal

Menopause-glandular

Vagal

Frontal eye fields

Temporal-emotional

B

Anterior fontanel

Frontal eye fields

Frontal-emotional

Anterior Pituitary

Extrinsic Eye muscles

Parotid gland

Maxillary sinus

Carotid sinus

Thyroid

Frontal eye fields

Frontal-emotional

Posterior pituitary

Extrinsic Eye muscles

Parotid gland

Maxillary sinus

Carotid sinus

Thyroid

Figure 5.9A,B,C Bennett's
C neurovascular reflex points.

Mobility tests form part of the diagnostic procedures in soft tissue assessment and since all manual therapists are concerned with joint mobility these tests will also be part of any overall assessment. Active motion, movement of one part of the body in relation to another, powered by conscious muscular effort as well as passive motion in which an outside force acts on the body to induce movement, are both of diagnostic importance. Eventually it is possible to rapidly distinguish between healthy tissue and tissue in which there exists dysfunction. This can only be learned by experience.

Observation, static and active; palpation, superficial and deep; a comprehensive and detailed history; mobility tests as required; localisation of trigger areas; re-evaluation during the course of treatment; and an intelligent cooperative understanding of the patient and his problems are the diagnostic tools with which to understand the task in hand.

Finding 'points' using NMT

Knowledge of Chapman's neurolymphatic areas, Bennett's reflexes, Mackenzie's reflex areas, connective tissue zones and trigger points might appear a massive task for the memory, and so it is. However, the application of the general knowledge of their existence enables treatment to be effective even without precise knowledge of all the individual reflexes involved. The aim of this chapter has been to try to classify some of the more obvious diagnostic indicators so that the practitioner's awareness can be broadened as to the range of diagnostic and therapeutic possibilities.

REFERENCES

Arbuckle B 1977 Selected writings. National Osteopathic Institute
Baldry P 1993 Acupuncture, trigger points and musculoskeletal pain. Churchill Livingstone, London
Beal M 1983 Palpatory testing of somatic dysfunction in patients with cardiovascular disease. Journal of the American Osteopathic Association July
Bischof I, Elmiger G 1960 Connective tissue massage. In: Licht E (ed) Massage, manipulation and traction. New Haven, Connecticut
Chaitow L 1965 An introduction to Chapman's reflexes. British Naturopathic Journal 6(4): 111–113
DiGiovanna E (ed) 1991 An osteopathic approach to diagnosis and treatment. Lippincott, Philadelphia
Koizumi K 1978 Autonomic system reactions, caused by excitation of somatic afferents: study of cutaneo-intestinal reflex. In: Korr I (ed) The Neurobiological Mechanisms in Manipulative Therapy
Lewit K 1992 Manipulative therapy in rehabilitation of the locomotor system. Butterworths, London

Lief P 1963 British Naturopathic Journal 5(10): 304–324
Mackenzie J 1909 Symptoms and their interpretations.
Owen F 1963 An endocrine interpretation of Chapman's reflexes. Academy of Applied Osteopathy
Speransky A 1943 A basis for the theory of medicine. International Publishers, New York
Stiles E 1984 Patient Care May 15 16–87 and 15 August 117–164
Teiriche-Leube H 1960 Grundriss der Bindesgewebsmassage. Fisher, Stuttgart
Travell J 1957 Symposium on mechanisms and management of pain syndromes. Proceedings Rudolph Virchow Medical Society
Travell J, Simons D 1983 Myofascial pain and dysfunction (vol 1) Williams and Wilkins
Travell J, Simons D 1992 Myofascial pain and dysfunction (vol 2) Williams and Wilkins
Youngs B 1964 NMT of lower thorax and low back. British Naturopathic Journal 5(11): 176–190, 340–358

6

Basic spinal NMT

DEFINING NMT

NMT, as the term is used in this book, is summarised in Box 6.1.

In this text the 'European' version of NMT, as developed by Stanley Lief, based partly on traditional Ayurvedic massage, has been described along with the subsequent evolution of American

---

Box 6.1   Aims of NMT and other allied approaches

- Neuromuscular technique, as the term is used in this book, refers to the manual application of specialised pressure and strokes, usually delivered by a finger or thumb contact, which have a diagnostic (assessment mode) or therapeutic (treatment mode) objective.
- Therapeutically, NMT aims to produce modifications in dysfunctional tissue, encouraging a restoration of normality, with a primary focus of deactivating focal points of reflexogenic activity such as myofascial trigger points.
- An alternative focus of NMT application is towards normalising imbalances in hypertonic and/or fibrotic tissues, either as an end in itself or as a precursor to joint mobilisation/rehabilitation.
- NMT utilises physiological responses involving neurological mechanoreceptors, golgi tendon organs, muscle spindles and other proprioceptors, in order to achieve the desired responses.
- Insofar as they integrate with NMT, other means of influencing such neural reporting stations, including positional release (strain/counterstrain) and muscle energy methods (such as reciprocal inhibition and postisometric relaxation induction) are seen to form a natural set of allied approaches.
- Traditional massage methods which encourage a reduction in retention of metabolic wastes and enhanced circulation to dysfunctional tissues are included in this category of allied approaches.

NMT methods, resulting from the work of Nimmo, St John and Walker, among others.

A confusing element relating to the term NMT emerges, due to its use by the Dvoraks, when they describe what are, in effect, variations on the theme of the use of isometric contractions in order to encourage a reduction in hypertonicity (Dvorak et al 1988). These methods, all of which form part of what is known as muscle energy technique (MET) in osteopathic medicine, are briefly described in Chapter 8 (p. 114), and form the focus of a further title in the series of which this book is part.

Dvorak's use of the terms NMT 1, 2 and 3 to describe these methods succeeds in adding to, rather than reducing, semantic confusion and it is hoped that this aberrant set of descriptions will not persist.

Dvorak has listed various MET methods (as NMT) as follows:

1. Methods which involve self mobilisation by patient action to encourage movement past a resistance barrier are called 'NMT 1' by Dvorak.

2. Isometric contraction and subsequent passive stretching of agonist muscles involving postisometric relaxation become 'NMT 2'.

3. Isometric contraction of antagonists, followed by stretching, involving reciprocal inhibition are called 'NMT 3' by Dvorak.

What is unique to NMT is its concentration on the soft tissues, not just to give reflex benefit to the body, not just to prepare for other therapeutic methods such as exercise or manipulation, not just to relax and normalise tense fibrotic muscular tissue and not just to enhance lymphatic and general circulation and drainage, but to do all these things and, at the same time, to be able to offer the practitioner diagnostic information via the palpating and treating instrument which is usually the thumb.

NMT can usefully be integrated in treatment aimed at postural reintegration, tension release, pain relief, improvement of joint mobility, reflex stimulation/modulation or sedation. There are many variations of the basic technique as developed by Stanley Lief the choice of which will depend upon particular presenting factors or personal preference. Similarities between some aspects of NMT and other manual systems (see Chapter 8, p. 124) should be anticipated, since techniques have been borrowed from other systems where appropriate.

NMT can be applied generally or locally and in a variety of positions (sitting, lying etc.). The order in which body areas are dealt with is not regarded as critical in general treatment but is of some consequence in postural reintegration.

The basic spinal NMT treatment and the basic abdominal (and related areas) NMT treatment are the most commonly used and will be described in detail in this and the next chapter. The methods described are in essence those of Stanley Lief and Boris Chaitow, both of whom achieved (and in the latter case continues to achieve) a degree of skill in the application of NMT that is unsurpassed. The inclusion of data on reflex areas and effects, together with basic NMT methods, provides the operator with a useful therapeutic tool, the limitations of which will be largely determined by the degree of intelligence and understanding with which it is employed. As Boris Chaitow has written (Chaitow 1983):

The important thing to remember is that this unique manipulative formula is applicable to any part of the body for any physical and physiological dysfunction and for both articular and soft tissue lesions.

To apply NMT successfully it is necessary to develop the art of palpation and sensitivity of fingers by constantly feeling the appropriate areas and assessing any abnormality in tissue structure for tensions, contractions, adhesions, spasms.

It is important to acquire with practice an appreciation of the 'feel' of normal tissue so that one is better able to recognise abnormal tissue. Once some level of diagnostic sensitivity with fingers has been achieved, subsequent application of the technique will be much easier to develop. The whole secret is to be able to recognise the 'abnormalities' in the feel of tissue structures. Having become accustomed to understanding the texture and character of 'normal' tissue, the pressure applied by the thumb in general, especially in the spinal structures, should always be firm, but never hurtful or bruising. To this end the pressure should be applied with a 'variable' pressure, i.e. with an appreciation of the texture and character of the tissue structures and according to the feel that sensitive fingers should have developed. The level of the pressure applied should not be consistent because the character and texture of tissue is always variable.

These variations can be detected by one's educated 'feel'. The pressure should, therefore, be so applied that the thumb is moved along its path of direction in a way which corresponds to the feel of the tissues.

This variable factor in finger pressure constitutes probably the most important quality an operator of NMT can learn, enabling him to maintain more effective control of pressure, develop a greater sense of diagnostic feel, and be far less likely to bruise the tissue.

THUMB CONSIDERATIONS

NMT thumb technique (Fig. 6.1)

Thumb technique as employed in NMT, in either assessment or treatment modes, enables a wide variety of therapeutic effects to be produced. The tip of the thumb can deliver varying degrees of pressure via any of four facets; the very tip may be employed or the medial or lateral aspect of the tip can be used to make contact with angled surfaces. For more general (less localised and less

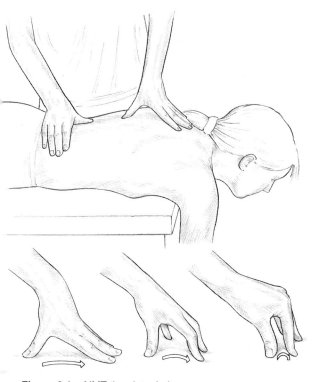

Figure 6.1   NMT thumb technique.

specific) contact, of a diagnostic or therapeutic type, the broad surface of the distal phalange of the thumb is often used. It is usual for a light, non-oily lubricant to be used to facilitate easy, non-dragging, passage of the palpating digit.

For balance and control the hand should be spread, tips of fingers providing a fulcrum or 'bridge' in which the palm is arched in order to allow free passage of the thumb towards one of the fingertips as the thumb moves in a direction which takes it away from the operator's body. During a single stroke, which covers between 2 and 3 inches (5–8 cm), the fingertips act as a point of balance while the chief force is imparted to the thumb tip via controlled application through the long axis of the extended arm of body weight. The thumb therefore never leads the hand but always trails behind the stable fingers, the tips of which rest just beyond the end of the stroke. Unlike many bodywork/massage strokes the hand and arm remain still as the thumb, applying variable pressure (see p. 92), moves through its pathway of tissue.

The extreme versatility of the thumb enables it to modify the direction of imparted force in accordance with the indications of the tissue being tested/treated. As the thumb glides across and through those tissues it becomes an extension of the operator's brain. In fact, for the clearest assessment of what is being palpated, the operator should have his eyes closed, in order that every minute change in the tissue can be felt and reacted to.

The thumb and hand seldom impart their own muscular force except in dealing with small localised contractures or fibrotic 'nodules'.

In order that pressure/force be transmitted directly to its target, the weight being imparted should travel in as straight a line as possible, which is why the arm should not be flexed at the elbow or the wrist by more than a few degrees. The positioning of the operator's body in relation to the area being treated is also of the utmost importance in order to facilitate economy of effort and comfort.

The optimum height *vis-à-vis* the couch, and the most effective angle of approach to the body areas being addressed, must be considered and the descriptions and illustrations will help to make this clearer.

The degree of pressure imparted will depend upon the nature of the tissue being treated, with a great variety of changes in pressure being possible during strokes across and through the tissues. When being treated, the patient should not feel strong pain but a general degree of discomfort is usually acceptable as the seldom stationary thumb varies its penetration of dysfunctional tissues. A stroke or glide of 2 to 3 inches (5–8 cm) will usually take 4 to 5 seconds, seldom more unless a particularly obstructive indurated area is being dealt with. If reflex pressure techniques are being employed, a much longer stay on a point will be needed, but in normal diagnostic and therapeutic use the thumb continues to move as it probes, decongests and generally treats the tissues.

It is not possible to state the exact pressures necessary in NMT application because of the very nature of the objective, which in assessment mode attempts to precisely meet and match the tissue resistance, to vary the pressure constantly in response to what is being felt.

In subsequent or synchronous (with assessment) treatment of whatever is uncovered during evaluation, a greater degree of pressure is used and this too will vary, depending upon the objective – whether this is to inhibit, to produce localised stretching, to decongest and so on. Obviously, on areas with relatively thin muscular covering, the applied pressure would be lighter than in tense or thick, well covered areas such as the buttocks.

Attention should also be paid to the relative sensitivity of different areas and different patients. The thumb should not just mechanically stroke across or through tissue but should become an intelligent extension of the operator's diagnostic sensitivities so that the contact feels to the patient as though it is sequentially assessing every important nook and cranny of the soft tissues. Pain should be transient and no bruising should result if the above advice is followed.

The treating arm and thumb should be relatively straight since a 'hooked' thumb, in which all the work is done by the distal phalange, will become extremely tired and will not achieve the degree of penetration possible via a fairly rigid thumb.

Hypermobile thumbs

Some operators have hypermobile joints and it is difficult for them to maintain sustained pressure without the thumb giving way and bending back on itself. This is a problem which can only be overcome by attempting to build up the muscular strength of the hand or by using a variation of the above technique, e.g. a knuckle or even the elbow may be used to achieve deep pressure in very tense musculature. Alternatively, the finger stroke as described below can take over from a hypermobile thumb.

NMT finger technique (Fig. 6.2)

In certain localities the width of the thumb prevents the degree of tissue penetration needed for successful assessment and/or treatment: in such

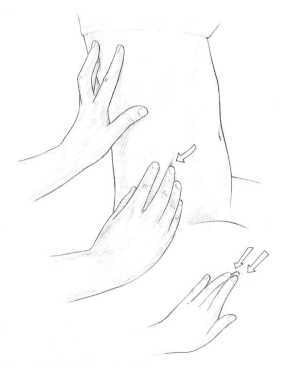

Figure 6.2   NMT finger technique.

regions the middle or index finger can usually be suitably employed. The most usual area for use of finger rather than thumb contact is in the intercostal musculature and in attempting to penetrate beneath the scapula borders in tense fibrotic conditions.

The middle or index finger should be slightly flexed and, depending upon the direction of the stroke and density of the tissues, supported by one of its adjacent members. As the treating finger strokes with a firm contact and usually a minimum of lubricant, a tensile strain is created between its tip and the tissue underlying it. This is stretched and lifted by the passage of the finger which, like the thumb, should continue moving unless or until dense, indurated tissue prevents its easy passage. These strokes can be repeated once or twice as tissue changes dictate.

The angle of pressure to the skin surface is between 40° and 50°. The fingertip should never lead the stroke but should always follow the wrist, the palmar surface of which should lead as the hand is drawn towards the operator. It is possible to impart a great degree of pull on underlying tissues and the patient's reactions must be taken into account in deciding on the degree of force to be used. Transient pain or mild discomfort are to be expected but no more than that. All sensitive areas are indicative of some degree of dysfunction, local or reflex, and are thus important, and their presence should be recorded. The patient should be told what to expect so that a cooperative, unworried attitude evolves.

Unlike the thumb technique, in which force is largely directed away from the operator's body, in finger treatment the motive force is usually towards the operator. The arm position therefore alters, and a degree of flexion is necessary to ensure that the pull or drag of the finger across the lightly lubricated tissues is smooth. Unlike the thumb, which makes a sweep towards the fingertips whilst the rest of the hand remains relatively stationary, the whole hand will move as finger pressure is applied. Certainly some variation in the degree of angle between fingertip and skin is allowable during a stroke and some slight variation in the degree of 'hooking'

of the finger is sometimes also necessary. However, the main motive force is applied by pulling the slightly flexed middle or index finger towards the operator with the possibility of some lateral emphasis if needed. The treating finger should always be supported by one of its neighbours.

Use of lubricant

The use of a lubricant to facilitate the smooth passage of, for example, the thumb over the surface is an essential aspect of NMT. The lubricant used should not allow too slippery a passage of the thumb or finger, and a suitable balance between lubrication and adherence is found by mixing 2 parts of rapeseed (or almond) oil to 1 part lime water. At times, the degree of stimulus imparted via this contact can be enhanced by increasing the tensile strain between the thumb or finger and the skin.

If this effect is required, notably to achieve a rapid vascular response, then no lubricant should be used. Clinical experience shows that similar reactions will be achieved (with lubricant) where NMT is applied along the intermuscular septa or at the origins and insertions of muscles.

It should be clear to the operator that underlying tissues being treated should be visualised and, depending upon the presenting symptoms and the area involved, any of a number of procedures may be undertaken as the hand moves from one site to another. There may be superficial stroking in the direction of lymphatic flow, or direct pressure along the line of axis of stress fibres, or deeper alternating 'make and break' stretching and pressure or traction on fascial tissue. As variable pressure is being applied, the operator needs to be constantly aware of diagnostic information which is being received via the contact hands and this is what determines the variations in pressure and the direction of force being applied. Any changes in direction or degree of applied pressure should ideally take place without any sudden release or application of force which could irritate the tissues and produce pain or a defensive contraction.

Lief's basic spinal treatment followed the pattern as set out below. The fact that the same pattern is followed at each treatment does not mean that the treatment is necessarily the same. The pattern gives a framework and a useful starting and ending point, but the degree of emphasis applied to the various areas of dysfunction that manifest themselves is a variable factor based always on what information the palpating hands are picking up: this is what makes each treatment different. The areas of dysfunction should be recorded on a case card, together with all relevant material and diagnostic findings relating to myofascial tissue changes, trigger points and reference zones, areas of sensitivity, restricted motion and so on.

LIEF'S BASIC SPINAL TREATMENT

Lief's basic spinal NMT treatment follows a pattern of placing the patient prone with a medium thickness pillow under the chest, forehead supported by the patient's hands or, ideally, resting in a split headpiece or face-hole. The whole spine from occiput to sacrum, including the gluteal area, is lightly oiled or creamed. The operator should begin by standing half-facing the head of the couch on the left of the patient, with his hips level with the mid-thoracic area. In order to facilitate the intermittent application of pressure and the transfer of weight via the arm to the exploring and treating thumb, the practitioner should stand with the left foot forward of the right by 12–18 inches (30–45 cm), weight evenly distributed between them, knees slightly flexed.

The first contact to the left side of the patient's head is a gliding, light-pressured movement of the medial tip of the right thumb, from the mastoid process along the nuchal line to the external occipital protuberance. This same stroke, or glide, is then repeated with deeper pressure.

The non-treating hand's role

The operator's left hand should at this time rest on the upper thoracic or shoulder area to act as a stabilising contact. Whichever hand is operating at any given time, the other hand can give assistance by means of gently rocking or stretching

tissues to complement the efforts of the treating hand, or it can be useful in distracting tissues which are 'mounding' as the treating hand works on them.

Whenever the operator changes to the other side of the table it is suggested that one hand always maintains light contact with the patient. Indeed, it is suggested that once treatment has commenced no breaks in contact be allowed. There is often a noticeable increase in tension in the tissues of the patient if the series of strokes, stretching movements and pressure techniques etc. which make up NMT is interrupted by even a few seconds because of a break in contact. Continuity would seem, in itself, to be of therapeutic value, simply as a reassuring and calming feature.

What the treating thumb feels

The movement of the right thumb through the tissue is slow – not uniformly slow, but deliberately seeking and feeling for 'contractions' and 'congestions' (to use two words which will be meaningful to any manual therapist). If and when such localised areas are felt, the degree of pressure can be increased and, in a variably applied manner, this pressure carries the thumb tip across or through the restricting tissues, decongesting, stretching and easing them.

The patient will often report a degree of pain but may say that it 'feels good'. It is a contradiction in terms, but constructive pain is usually felt as a 'nice hurt'.

Practitioner's posture (Fig. 6.3)

The treating arm should not be flexed, since the optimum transmission of weight from the operator's shoulder, through the arm to the thumb tip, is best achieved with a relatively straight arm. This demands that the practitioner ensures that the table height is suitable for his own height. He should not be forced to stand on tiptoe to treat his patient, nor should he have to adopt an unhealthy bent posture. The operator's weight should be evenly spread between the

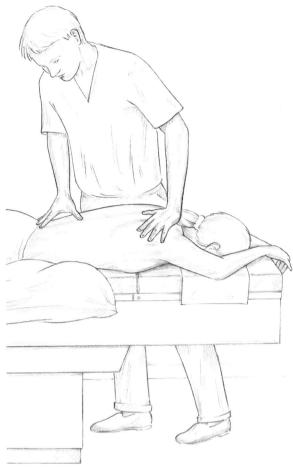

Figure 6.3 NMT – operator's posture should ensure a straight treating arm for ease of transmission of body weight, as well as leg positions which allow for the easy transfer of weight and the centre of gravity. These postures assist in reducing energy expenditure and ease spinal stress.

separated feet, both of which are forward facing at this stage. In this way, by slightly altering his own weight distribution from the front to the back foot, and vice versa, an accurate, controlled degree of pressure can be exerted with minimum arm or hand effort.

Weight transfer – key to economy of effort

The hand itself should not be rigid but in a relaxed state, moulding itself to the contours of the neck or back tissues. To some extent the

fingertips stabilise the hand. The thumb's glide is controlled by this, so that the actual stroke is achieved by the tip of the extended thumb being brought slowly across the palm towards the fingertips. The fingers, during this phase of cervical treatment, would be placed on the opposite side of the neck to that being treated. The fingers maintain their position as the thumb performs its diagnostic/therapeutic glide. The illustrations will aid the reader to a better understanding of this description (see Fig 6.4A,B).

However, were all the effort to be on the part of the thumb it would soon tire. Consider which parts of the operator's arm/hand are involved with the various aspects of the glide/stroke as delivered by the thumb (finger strokes involve completely different mechanics):

- The transverse movement of the thumb is a hand or forearm effort.
- The relative straightness or rigidity of the last two thumb segments is also a local muscular responsibility.
- The vast majority of the energy imparted via the thumb results from transmission of body weight through the straight arm and into the thumb.
- Any increase in pressure can be speedily achieved by simple weight transfer from back towards front foot and a slight 'lean' onto the thumb from the shoulders.
- A lessening of imparted pressure is achieved by reversing this body movement.

The first two strokes of the right thumb having been completed – one shallow and almost totally diagnostic and the second, deeper, imparting therapeutic effort – the next stroke is half a thumb width caudal to the first. Thus a degree of overlap occurs as these strokes, starting on the belly of the sternocleidomastoid, glide across and through the trapezius, splenius capitus and posterior cervical muscles. A progressive series of strokes is applied in this way until the level of the cervicodorsal junction is reached. Unless serious underlying dysfunction is found it is seldom necessary to repeat the two superimposed strokes at each level of the cervical region.

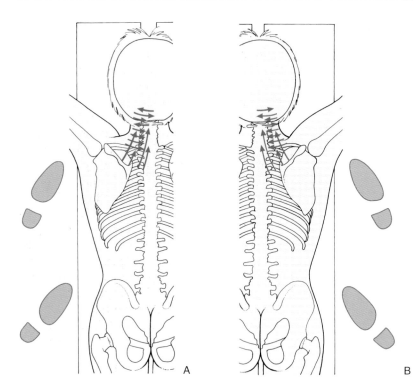

Figure 6.4A,B First positions of suggested sequence of applications of NMT, to ensure optimal thumb and/or finger contact with primary trigger point sites and with the origins and insertions of most muscles. Note foot positions.

Variable pressure – the key to painless pressure

If underlying fibrotic tissue appears unyielding a third or fourth slow, deep glide may be necessary. The degree of discomfort felt by the patient is of some importance. The sensitivity of this region is well known and if pressure is too deep, or sustained too long, the defensive resistance that may be created can make the treatment counterproductive. It is possible to achieve deep, penetrating pressure, if it is variable in nature and not long held, without undue pain or discomfort. Thus a thinking, intuitive feel for the work is a prerequisite of successful application. Should trigger points be located, as indicated by the reproduction in a target area of an existing pain pattern, then a number of choices are open:[1]

1. The point can be marked and noted (on a chart and if necessary on the body with a skin pencil).

2. Sustained pressure or 'make and break' pressure can be used (see Ch. 8, p. 113).

3. Application of a positional release approach (strain/counterstrain) will reduce activity in the hyper-reactive tissue, as outlined in Chapter 8 (p. 131).

4. Initiation of an isometric contraction followed by stretch could be used.

5. A combination of pressure, positional release and MET (INIT) can be introduced, as discussed in Chapter 8 (p. 114) and more fully in Chapter 9 (p. 137).

6. Spray and stretch methods can be used (vapocoolant technique as discussed in Chapter 8, p. 110).

7. An acupuncture needle or a procaine injection can be used.

Sustained pressure, if applied, should be slightly variable i.e., deep pressure for 5 to 7 seconds followed by a slight easing for a further few

---

[1]Whichever approach is used, a trigger point will only be permanently deactivated if the muscle in which it lies is restored to its normal resting length, and MET can assist in achieving this.

seconds and so on, repeated until the reference pain diminishes or until the maximum time (2 minutes) has elapsed. No more than this amount of manual pressure should be applied to a trigger point at any one session.

Further ease of the hyper-reactive patterns in a trigger point can be achieved by applying ultrasound (pulsed) or by the application of a hot towel to the area, followed by effleurage.

The neck treatment continues

Once the right thumb has completed its series of transverse strokes across the long axis of the cervical musculature, the left hand, which has been resting on the patient's left shoulder, now comes into play. A series of strokes is applied by the left thumb, upward from the left of the upper dorsal area towards the base of the skull. The fingers of the left hand rest (and act as a fulcrum) on the front of the shoulder area at the level of the medial aspect of the clavicle. The thumb tip should be angled to allow direct pressure to be exerted against the left lateral aspects of the upper dorsal and the lower cervical spinous processes as the thumb glides cephalid. The subsequent strokes of the thumb should be in the same direction but slightly more laterally placed. The fingers should then be placed on the patient's head at about the temporooccipital articulation. The left thumb then deals in the same way with the mid and upper cervical soft tissues, finishing with a lateral stroke or two across the insertions on the occiput itself.

In travelling from the nuchal line to the level of the cervicodorsal junction and back again in a series of overlapping gliding movements, common sites of a number of possible trigger points will have been evaluated. The mid-point of the sternomastoid, at the level of the posterior angle of the jaw, can be a source of intensely painful trigger which refers its influence from the area above the temple in the ear region to below the angle of the jaw. Similar triggers exist in the splenius capitus, upper trapezius, posterior cervical and other muscles of the area, all with different target areas.

Posterior reflex centres

Also in this area there occur the posterior reflex centres of the neurolymphatic type (Chapman's reflexes), notably those connected with conjunctivitis, cerebellar congestion and ear, nose and throat problems of an inflammatory or congested type, from sinusitis to tonsillitis. It is suggested that due study is made of the illustrations of neurolymphatic reflex positions (p. 79). Treatment of these points is via lightly sustained pressure, as described in Chapter 4 (p. 53).

Recall at this point that Gutstein (Ch. 3, p. 28) found trigger areas in the cervical and upper dorsal region which profoundly affected such diverse conditions as menopausal symptoms, imbalance in skin secretions and excessive perspiration. He stressed the importance of the cervical region and the interscapular area.

Among the more important *Tsubo* or acupressure points in the upper cervical area are:

- Gall bladder 20, which lies bilaterally in a depression midway between the occipital protuberance and the mastoid at the base of the skull
- Bladder 10, which lies bilaterally just lateral to the large bundle of muscular insertions at the occiput
- Triple heater 17, which lies bilaterally in the depression between the lobe of ear and the mastoid process.

These points, if sensitive, should receive a sustained or variable pressure, as for the other trigger points. Their influence is felt in a variety of conditions relating to the head, such as migraine, neuralgia, cold symptoms, hyper- and hypotension, liver dysfunction etc.

Goodheart (1987) mentions levator scapulae 'weakness' as indicating digestive problems and recommends pressure techniques in the cervicodorsal area and on the medial border of the scapula to help normalise this.

Following the treatment of the left side of the cervical area the same procedures are repeated on the right. A tall operator can probably adapt to treat both sides of the area from one standing position; however, a move to the opposite side makes for a more controlled delivery of the appropriate strokes.

Origins and insertions

During NMT treatment special notice should be given to the origins and insertions of the muscles of the area. Where these bony landmarks are palpable by the thumb tip they should be treated by the slow, variably applied pressure technique. Indeed, all bony surfaces within reach of the probing digit should be searched for undue sensitivity and dysfunction of their attachments, which are amongst the commonest sites of trigger points according to Travell.

How long?

Treatment of the left cervical area should take no more than 2 minutes and, in the absence of dysfunction, can be comfortably and success- fully dealt with in 90 seconds, or less. Indeed, in its assessment mode, the entire basic spinal NMT treatment can usually be completed in 15 minutes.

Adopting a new position

Once both left and right cervical areas have been treated, the operator moves to the head of the table (Fig. 6.5). Resting the tips of the fingers on the lower, lateral aspect of the patient's neck, the thumb tips are placed just lateral to the first dorsal– spinal process. A degree of downward (towards the floor) pressure is applied via the thumbs, which are then drawn cephalid along- side the lateral margins of the cervical spinous processes. This bilateral stroke culminates at the occiput, where a lateral stretch or pull is intro- duced across the bunched fibres of the muscles inserting into the base of the skull.

The upward stroke should contain an element of pressure medially towards the spinous pro- cess, so that the pad of the thumb is pressing downward (towards the floor) whilst the lateral thumb tip is directed towards the centre, attempt- ing to contact the bony contours of the spine, all the time being drawn slowly cephalid to end at the occiput. This combination stroke is repeated

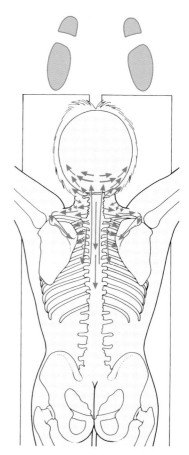

Figure 6.5 Third position of suggested sequence of application of NMT.

two or three times. The fingertips which have been resting on the sternomastoid may also be employed at this stage, to lift and stretch it pos- teriorly and laterally. The lateral stretch across the occipital protuberance may be likened to trying to break open a melon. The thumb tips dig deep into the medial fibres of the paraocci- pital bundle and an outward stretch is instituted, using the leverage of the arms, as though attempt- ing to open out the occiput. The thumbs are then drawn laterally across the fibres of muscular insertion into the skull, in a series of strokes cul- minating at the occipitoparietal junction.

The fingertips which act as a fulcrum to these movements rest on the mastoid area of the tem- poral bone. Several strokes are then performed by one thumb or the other running caudad

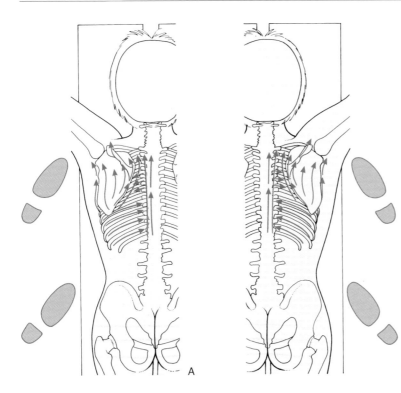

Figure 6.6A,B Fourth (A) and fifth (B) positions of suggested sequence of applications of NMT.

directly over the spinous process from the base of the skull to the upper dorsal area. Pressure should be moderate and slow. Standing in the same position, the left thumb will now be placed on the right, lateral aspect of the first dorsal vertebra and a series of strokes are performed caudad and laterally as well as diagonally towards the scapula.

The fingers should be splayed out ahead of the thumb in whichever direction it is travelling, so that the force transmitted via the extended arm can be controlled. The fingers act as a fulcrum, with the thumb tip being drawn across the palm towards the diagonally opposite point – the tip of the middle or little finger. The thumb should never lead the hand nor be solely 'digging' or pressing without the stabilising and controlling action of the hand or fingertips also being in operation.

A series of strokes, shallow and then deep, is therefore applied from D1 to about D4 or 5 and outwards towards the scapula and along and across the upper trapezius fibres and the rhom-boids. The left hand treats the right side, and vice versa, with the nonoperative hand resting on the neck or head stabilising it. Weight transfer to the thumb is achieved as described previously, by leaning forward.

Trapezius and sternomastoid muscles

Standing at the head of the table facing caudad allows the operator to access the region of the upper trapezius from above, so to speak. By lowering the angle at which the hand contacts the muscle, perhaps by kneeling or at least by lowering the centre of gravity significantly, and by standing a little to one side of the centre, it is possible to apply a series of sensitively searching contacts into the area of the thoracic outlet. Strokes which start in this triangular depression would move towards the trapezius fibres and through them towards the upper margins of the scapula. A treasure house of trigger points awaits this searching digit.

Since it is often difficult to apply pressure to the trapezius or sternomastoid muscles in such a way as to involve underlying bony structures it may be necessary to lightly pinch or squeeze the more sensitive areas of dysfunction to assess trigger points and their related target areas of pain. Several strokes should also be applied directly over the spinous processes caudad as far down as the mid-dorsal area. Triggers sometimes lie on the attachments to the spinous processes or between them.

By referring to the illustrations of trigger points (pp xiii–xv) the location of the commonest trigger points can be predicted and their presence rapidly established. When it is not possible to apply thumb pressure to such a point, a squeezing of the involved muscle area instead of direct pressure into it, again using varying pressure as described above (p. 94), will usually induce a reduction of the referred pain. Once pain reduces, the pressure should be released. If no success is achieved by these means then one of the other approaches outlined can be used.

Left side trunk treatment

The operator then moves to the patient's left side and stands in the same manner as at the commencement of the treatment but at the level of the patient's waist. With the right hand now resting at the level of the lower dorsal spine, the left thumb commences a series of strokes cephalid from the mid-dorsal area. Each stroke covers two or three spinal segments and runs immediately lateral to the spinous process so that the angle of pressure imparted via the medial tip of the thumb is roughly towards the contralateral nipple. Again, light assessment and deep therapeutic strokes are employed and a degree of overlap is allowed on successive strokes.

In this way the first two strokes might run from D8 to D5 followed by two strokes (one light, one deeper) from D6 to D3 and finally two strokes from D4 to D1. Deeper and more sustained pressure can be exerted upon discovering marked congestion or resistance to the gliding, probing thumb. In the dorsal area a second line of upward strokes may be employed to include

the spinal border of the scapula as well as one or two searching lateral probes along the inferior spine of the scapula and across the musculature inferior to and inserting into the scapula (see Fig. 6.6A).

Right side treatment

Treatment of the right side may be carried out without necessarily changing position, other than to lean across the patient. However, the shorter practitioner should change sides so that, standing half-facing the head of the patient, the right thumb can perform the strokes discussed above. Apart from trigger points in the lower trapezius fibres others may be sought in levator scapulae, supra- and infraspinatus, and subscapularis (by accessing via the axilla). The connective tissue zones affecting the arm, stomach, heart, liver and gall bladder are apparent in the region now being treated and neurolymphatic reflexes relating to the arm, thyroid, lungs, throat and heart occur in the upper dorsal spine, including the scapular area.

The intercostal spaces are a rich site of dysfunction. The thumb tip or a fingertip should be run along both surfaces of the rib margin as well as in the intercostal space itself. In this way the fibres of the small muscles involved will be adequately treated. If there is over approximation of the ribs then a simple stroke along the space may be all that is possible until a degree of normalisation has taken place. These intercostal areas are extremely sensitive and care must be taken not to distress the patient. In most instances the intercostal spaces on the side opposite that on which the operator is standing will be treated using the finger stroke, as illustrated (Fig. 6.6A,B).

The tip of a finger is placed in the intercostal space and gently but firmly brought upwards and around the curve of the trunk towards the spine, feeling for contracted or congested tissues in which trigger points might be located.

Change of position

The practitioner now half turns so that instead of facing the patient's head he faces the patient's *[handwritten margin notes at top:]* Rhomboid weakness indicates liver problems! C7 pressure ... point on the RT side of the ... interspace between dorsal spinous processes 5+6 assist ... TS NORMAL

feet. The pattern of strokes is now carried out on the patient's left side by the operator's right hand (Fig. 6.7). A series starting from D8 to D11, followed by D 11 to L 1 and then L 1 to L4, is carried out as before. Two or more gliding strokes with the pressure downwards but angled so that the medial aspect of the thumb is in contact with the lateral margin of the spinous process, are performed at each level.

The lower intercostal areas are treated as described above. The operator steps back from the table and glides the thumb to allow access to a stroke which runs along the superior iliac spine from just above the hip to the sacroiliac joint. Several such strokes may be applied into the heavy musculature above the crest of ilium. To treat the opposite side, the operator changes sides so that he is facing the patient's waist and half-turned towards the feet; the left hand can deal with the lower dorsal and upper lumbar area and the iliac crest in the manner described above. One or two strokes should then be applied running caudad over the tips of the spinous processes from the mid-dorsal area to the sacrum.

The area we have been describing contains a network of reflex areas and points. The *Tsubo* or acupressure points lying symmetrically on either side of the spine and along the midline have great reflex importance. The so-called 'Bladder meridian' points lie in two lines running parallel with the spine, one level with the medial border of the scapula and the other midway between it and the lateral border of the spinous processes. Goodheart's work (1987) suggests that rhomboid weakness indicates liver problems and that pressure on C7 spinous process and a point on the right of the interspace between the fifth and sixth dorsal spinous process assists its normalisation. Latissimus dorsi weakness apparently indicates pancreatic dysfunction. Lateral to seventh and eighth dorsal interspace is the posterior pressure reflex to normalise this. These and other reflexes would appear to derive from Chapman's reflex theories and are deserving of further study.

[handwritten margin notes:] Liver Prob.

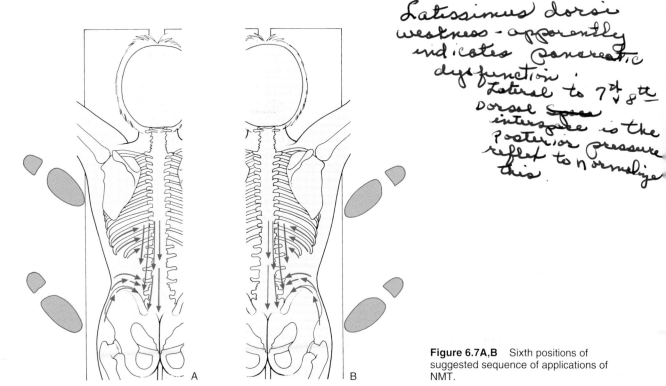

[handwritten note beside figure:] Latissimus dorsi weakness - apparently indicates pancreatic dysfunction. Lateral to 7th & 8th Dorsal Space interspace is the Posterior pressure reflex to normalize this.

Figure 6.7A,B   Sixth positions of suggested sequence of applications of NMT.

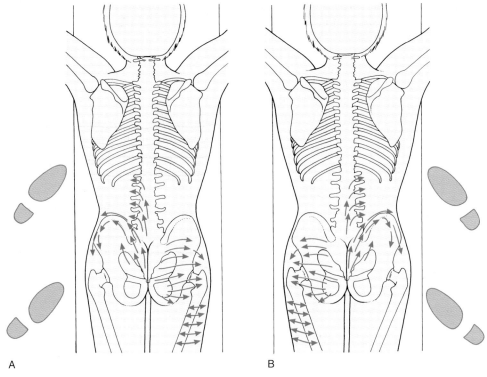

A   B

Figure 6.8A,B Seventh positions of suggested sequence of applications of NMT.

In general terms, dysfunction of the erector spinae group of muscles, between sixth and twelfth dorsal, indicates liver involvement. Similarly fourth, fifth and sixth dorsal area congestion or sensitivity usually involves stomach reflexes and gastric disturbance, whereas D12 and L2 indicates possible kidney dysfunction.

Left hip position

The next treatment position requires the operator to stand at the level of the patient's left hip, half-facing the head of the couch. The left hand and thumb describe a series of cephalad strokes from the sacral apex towards the sacroiliac area, and then laterally along the superior and inferior margins of the iliac crest to the insertion of the tensor fascia lata at the anterior, superior iliac spine (Fig. 6.8). A further series of short strokes of the thumb upwards and laterally in the lumbar area are best described as attempting to

stretch and open out from the spine the muscles of the area, notably the sacrospinal group.

Having treated both left and right sides of the lumbar spine as above the operator uses a series of two-handed gliding manoeuvres in which the hands are spread over the upper gluteal area laterally, the thumb tips are placed at the level of the second sacral foramen with a downward (towards the floor) pressure; they glide cephalid and slowly laterally to pass over and through the fibres of the sacroiliac joint. This is repeated several times.

Still standing on the left, the operator leans across the patient's upper thigh and engages his right thumb onto the ischial tuberosity. A series of gliding movements are carried out from that point laterally to the hip and caudad towards the gluteal fold. A further series of strokes, always applying deep, probing, but variable pressure is then carried out from the sacral border across the gluteal area to the hip margins. The fingertips during these strokes are splayed out so that they can guide and balance the hand and thumb movement. In these deep muscles the line of the thumb's direction is more towards the tip of the index finger or middle finger rather than to the little fingertip, as it was in the cervical area. In deep, tense gluteal muscle the thumb can be inadequate to the task of prolonged pressure techniques and the elbow may be used to sustain deep pressure for minutes at a time. Care should be taken, however, as the degree of pressure possible by this means is enormous and tissue damage and bruising can result from its careless employment.

The operator moves to the right side and repeats the same strokes.

Alternatively, rather than changing sides the operator can lean across the patient and use hooked finger strokes to effectively access the tissues above the hip and around the curve of the iliac crest.[2]

Having treated the low lumbar area and the gluteals, the operator might usefully include a series of strokes across the fibres of the tensor fascia lata from the hip area to the lateral knee area. The tensor fascia lata contains neurolymphatic reflexes to the groin glands, the broad ligaments, spastic constipation and colitis, prostate etc. and is itself a major contributor to knee, pelvic and low back problems via its influence on the mechanics of the region. It is commonly extremely sensitive to pressure and care is needed to prevent patient distress in treating it.

Completion of treatment

This completes the basic spinal NMT treatment apart from any manipulative procedures that might be indicated or thought desirable. Boris Chaitow completes the spinal treatment by standing at the head of the table, leaning over the patient's upper dorsal area, the palms of both

---

[2]Trigger points, connective tissue zones and neurolymphatic reflexes that may be involved in the lower lumbar and gluteal areas are shown in Box 6.2.

Box 6.2 Trigger points, connective tissue zones and neurolymphatic reflexes of the lower lumbar and gluteal areas

- The trigger points that may be found in the lower lumbar and gluteal areas include those in the following muscle groups: iliocostal, multifidus, longissimus, gluteus medius and gluteus minimus.
- The connective tissue zones that may be involved include those that involve arterial and venous disturbance to the legs, constipation, liver, gall bladder, heart and bladder.
- The neurolymphatic reflexes include those that involve the following areas and conditions: the appendix, haemorrhoids, female generative organs, vasiculitis, sciatic nerve, abdominal tension and constipation, prostate, colitis, kidneys, adrenal glands, digestive system, pancreas, liver, spleen and gall bladder.

hands totally in contact with the upper lumbar region so that the thenar eminence is resting on the paraspinal musculature and the fingers pointing laterally. The heel of the hand imparts the main contact laterally. A series of gliding strokes is performed with the hands rhythmically alternating with each other so that as the right hand strokes downwards to end its movement on the gluteals the left is being brought back to the lower dorsal area. After it descends the right hand comes back to the start. In this way a series of ten to twenty deep rhythmic strokes are carried out in order to stimulate local circulation and drainage as well as to further relax the patient, who may well have tensed during the treatment of the lumbar and gluteal areas. As stated previously, the basic 'assessment' treatment should take no more than 15 minutes; however, far longer may be needed if whatever is found of a dysfunctional nature is treated.

The patient should have a sense of release from tension and a sense of well being which may last for some days. Many feel a sense of tiredness and a great desire to sleep; this should be encouraged. Pain may result in those areas that have borne the main brunt of the pressure techniques and this should be explained to the patient, who should be encouraged to note any changes in her condition and to report these at the subsequent visit. The frequency of application of NMT will vary with the condition. In chronic conditions one or two treatments weekly are as much as is ever required. This can be maintained until progress dictates that the interval be lengthened.

In acute conditions treatment may be much more frequent: daily if possible until ease is achieved. Of necessity, this must depend upon what other modalities are employed.

REFERENCES

Chaitow B 1983 Personal communication to the author.
Dvorak J, Dvorak V, Schneider W 1988 Manual medicine therapy. Georg Thieme Verlag, Stuttgart
Goodheart G 1987 Applied kinesiology workshop procedure manuals 1976–1987. Published privately, Detroit
Travell J, Simons D 1986 Myofascial pain and dysfunction. Williams & Wilkins, Baltimore

7

Basic abdominal NMT application

AREAS FOR TREATMENT

In treating the abdominal and related areas our attention should focus on specific junctional tissues. These comprise the central tendon and the lateral aspect of the rectal muscle sheaths, the insertion of the recti muscles and external oblique muscles into the ribs, the xiphisternal ligament as well as the lower insertions of the internal and external oblique muscles. The intercostal areas from fifth to twelfth ribs are equally important. Specific general areas are worthy of consideration in treating conditions affecting particular organs or functions based on the evidence of the different reflex 'systems' described in Chapter 4 (p. 49):

- Liver dysfunction and portal circulatory dysfunction would call for special attention to the right side intercostal musculature from fifth to twelfth ribs. Especially important are the various muscular insertions into all these ribs.
- Gall bladder dysfunction involves the above areas with extra attention to the area on the costal margin, roughly midway between the xiphisternal notch and the lateral rib margins.
- Spleen function may be stimulated by attention to the intercostal spaces between the seventh and twelfth ribs on the left side.
- Digestive disorders in general will benefit from NMT applied to the central tendon between the recti and directly to the rectal sheaths.
- Stomach pain is treated via its reflex area to the left of the xiphisternal notch and to the tendon and rectal sheaths.

- Colonic problems and ovarian dysfunction will benefit from reflex NMT application to both iliac fossae as well as to the midline structures.
- Dysfunction of the kidneys, ureters and bladder require attention to the inguinal borders of the internal and external oblique insertions, the suprapubic insertions of the recti, the overlying muscles and sheaths of the area and the internal aspects of the upper thigh.
- In pelvic congestion relating to gynaecological dysfunction, NMT should be applied to the hypogastrium and both iliac fossae. This relieves congestion and stimulates pelvic circulation.
- Ileitis and other functional disturbances of the transverse colon and small intestine benefit from NMT applied to the umbilical area.
- Prostatic dysfunction will benefit from NMT to the central hypogastric region. Internal drainage massage of the prostate should also be considered.

The above brief indications should be considered in conjunction with other reflex systems and points (see below) as well as attention to the appropriate spinal areas (see notes on facilitation in Chapter 3, p. 30) which would also benefit from NMT treatment.

ABDOMINAL REFLEX AREAS

Gutstein (1944) has noted trigger areas in the sternal, parasternal and epigastric regions and the upper portions of the rectus, all relating to varying degrees of retroperistalsis. He also noted that colonic dysfunction related to triggers in the mid and lower rectus muscle. These were all predominantly left-sided. Other symptoms which improved or disappeared with the obliteration of these triggers include excessive appetite, poor appetite, flatulence, nervous vomiting, nervous diarrhoea etc. The triggers were always tender spots, easily found by the palpation and situated mainly in the upper, mid and lower portions of the recti muscles, over the lower portion of the sternum and the epigastrium including the xyphoid process and the parasternal regions. The

parasternal region corresponds to the insertions of the rectus muscle into the fifth, sixth and seventh ribs.

Fielder (Fielder & Pyott 1955) described a number of reflexes occurring on the large bowel itself. These could be localised by deep palpation and treated by specific release techniques. These reflexes palpate as areas of tenderness and may include a degree of swelling and congestion resulting from adhesions, spasticity, diverticuli, chemical or bacterial irritation etc.

In considering the reflexes available in the thoracic and abdominal regions, the neurolymphatic points of Chapman are also worthy of close attention.[1] To what extent Gutstein's myodysneuric points are interchangeable with Chapman's reflexes or Fielder's reflexes, or other systems of reflex study (e.g. acupuncture or *Tsubo* points and Travell's triggers) and to what extent these involve Mackenzie's work (Mackenzie 1909) is a matter for further research.[1]

What is certain is that within the soft tissues of this region there abound palpable, sensitive, discrete areas of dysfunction which, on a local basis, interfere with or modify functional integrity to a greater or lesser degree, and reflexively are capable of massive interference with normal physiological function on a neural, circulatory and lymphatic level, to the extent of producing or mimicking serious pathological conditions. Since these areas of dysfunction will often yield to the simple, soft tissue manipulative techniques which are incorporated into Lief's NMT, the value of these techniques becomes apparent.

Many of Jones's tender points are found in the abdominal regions specifically relating to those strains which occur in a flexed position (Jones 1981). Bennett's neurovascular points (see Ch. 4, p. 51) are mainly located on the anterior aspect of the body and may be located during abdominal NMT work. This may be a link with the work of Mackenzie and others, who demonstrated a clear relationship between the abdominal wall and the viscera. This and other reflex patterns

---

[1]Refer to Reference list in Chapter 4 (p. 63) for citations.

provide the rationale for NMT application to the abdominal and sternal regions. These reflex patterns vary in individual cases but it is clear that the majority of the organs are able to protect themselves by producing contraction, spasm and hyperaesthesia of the overlying, reflexively related muscle wall – the myotome – which is also often augmented by hyperaesthesia of the overlying skin – the dermatome.

Baldry (1993) details a huge amount of research which validates the link (a somatovisceral reflex) between abdominal trigger points and symptoms as diverse as anorexia, flatulence, nausea, vomiting, diarrhoea, colic, dysmenorrhoea and dysuria. Pain of a deep aching nature, or sometimes of a sharp or burning type are reported as being associated with this range of symptoms, which mimic organ disease or dysfunction (Hoyt 1953, Melnick 1954, Ranger et al 1971, Theobald, 1949, Travell & Simons 1983). Baldry (1993) has further summarised the importance of this region as a source of considerable pain and distress involving pelvic, abdominal and gynaecological symptoms. He says:

Pain in the abdomen and pelvis most likely to be helped by acupuncture is that which occurs as a result of activation of trigger points in the muscles, fascia, tendons and ligaments of the anterior and lateral abdominal wall, the lower back, the floor of the pelvis and the upper anterior part of the thigh. Such pain, however, is all too often erroneously assumed to be due to some intra-abdominal lesion, and as a consequence of being inappropriately treated is often allowed to persist for much longer than is necessary.

If we replace the word acupuncture with the term 'appropriate manual methods' we can come to appreciate that a large amount of abdominal and pelvic distress is remediable via the methods outlined in this book.

What activates these triggers? Similar factors as produce 'stress' anywhere else in the musculo-skeletal system – postural faults, trauma, environmental stressors such as cold and damp, surgery (another form of trauma) and so on. Differential diagnosis is obviously important in a region housing so many vital organs, and attention to the overall pattern of symptom presentation is critical. If in doubt get expert opinion.

Is the pain in the muscle or an organ?

Since there is no underlying osseous structure available to allow compression of the musculature of much or the soft tissues of the abdomen there is a need for a particular strategy which helps to screen palpated pain occurring at depth from that being produced in surface tissues.

When a local area of pain is noted using NMT or any other palpation method it should be firmly compressed by the palpating digit, sufficient to produce pain/referred pain (if a trigger is involved) but not enough to cause distress. The supine patient is then asked to raise both (straight) legs from the table (heels must be raised several inches). As this happens there will be a contraction of the abdominal muscles which produces a compression of the trigger point between the muscle and the finger/thumb and pain should increase. If pain decreases on the raising of the legs the site of the pain is beneath the muscle and probably involves a visceral problem.

It is of course possible for there to be a problem in the viscera and in the abdominal wall, in which case this test would be in error in ascribing all symptoms of pain to a muscle wall lesion. The test therefore gives a clue but not an absolute finding.

ABDOMINAL NMT APPLICATION

In treating the abdominal and thoracic regions the patient should be supine with the head supported by a medium-sized pillow and the knees flexed, either with a bolster under them or drawn right up so that the feet approximate the buttocks. Generous application of lubricant should be made to the area being treated.

Intercostal treatment

The operator is positioned to be level with the patient's waist and a series of strokes is applied with the tip of the thumb along the course of the intercostal spaces from the sternum, laterally. It is important that the insertions of the internal and external muscles receive attention. The margins of the ribs, both inferior and superior aspects, should receive firm gliding pressure from the distal phalanx of the thumb or middle finger.

If there is too little space to allow such a degree of differentiated pressure then a simple stroke along the available intercostal space suffices.

If the thumb cannot be insinuated between the ribs a finger (side of finger) contact can be used in which this is drawn towards the operator from the side opposite the one on which she is standing, up to the sternum.

The intercostals from the fifth rib to the costal margin are given a series of two or three deep, slow-moving, gliding, sensitive strokes on each side with special reference to points of particular congestion or sensitivity. These areas may benefit from up to 30 seconds of sustained or variable pressure techniques.

These points will not bear heavy pressure such as may be required in more heavily muscled regions and caution is called for. The operator should bear in mind the various reflex patterns in the region. Gentle probing on the sternum itself may elicit sensitivity in the rudimentary sternalis muscle which has been found to house trigger points. If this is found to be sensitive then any of the various trigger point treatments recommended in Chapter 8 may be used.

It is not necessary for the operator to change sides during the treatment of the intercostals unless it is found to be more comfortable to do so.

The operator should be facing the patient and be half-turned towards the head with legs apart for an even distribution of weight and with knees flexed to facilitate the transfer of pressure through the arms. Since many of the manoeuvres in the intercostal area and on the abdomen itself involve finger and thumb movements of a lighter nature than those applied through the heavy spinal musculature, the elbows need not be kept so straight.

However, when deep pressure is called for, and especially when this is applied via the thumb, the same criterion of weight transference from the shoulder through the thumb applies and the straightish arm is then an advantage for the economic and efficient use of energy.

Having treated the intercostal musculature and connective tissue and having dealt with any trigger points that have been found, the operator, using either a deep thumb pressure or a contact with the pads of the fingertips, applies a series of short strokes in a combination of oblique lateral and inferior directions from the xyphoid process.

Rectal sheath

This is followed by the same contact in a series of deep slow strokes along and under the costal margins. A series of short strokes with fairly deep but not painful pressure is then applied by the thumb, from the midline up to the lateral rectal sheath. This series of strokes starts just inferior to the xyphoid and concludes at the pubic promontory. The series may be repeated on each side several times, depending upon the degree of tension, congestion and sensitivity.

A similar pattern of treatment is followed across the lateral border of the rectal sheath. A

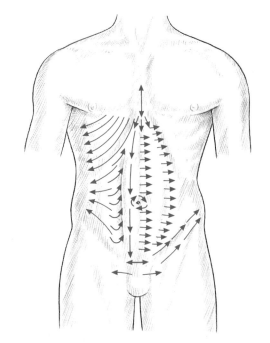

Figure 7.1 Neuromuscular abdominal technique. Suggested lines of application to access primary trigger point and attachment sites, and interfaces between different muscle groups.

series of short, deep, slow-moving thumb strokes being applied from just inferior to the costal margin of the rectal sheath until the inguinal ligament is reached. Both sides are treated in this way (Fig. 7.1).

A series of similar strokes is then applied on the one side and then the other laterally from the lateral border of the rectal sheath. These strokes follow the contour of the trunk so that the upper strokes travel in a slightly inferior curve whilst passing laterally and the lower strokes have a superior inclination, as the hand passes laterally. A total of five or six strokes would be adequate to complete these movements and this could be repeated before performing the same movements on the opposite side.

In treating the side on which the operator is standing it may be more comfortable to apply the therapeutic stroke via the flexed finger tips which are drawn towards the operator, or the usual thumb stroke may be used. In treating the opposite side, thumb pressure can more easily be applied, as in spinal technique, with the fingers acting as a fulcrum and the thumb gliding towards them in a series of 2 or 3 inch-long strokes. The sensing of contracted, gangliform areas of dysfunction is more difficult in abdominal work and requires great sensitivity of touch and great concentration on the part of the operator.

Symphysis pubis

Attention should be given to the insertions into, and the soft tissue component of, the pubic bones and the symphysis pubis. A deep but not painful stroke, employing the pad of the thumb, should be applied to the superior aspect of the pubic crest. This should start at the symphysis pubis and move laterally, first in one direction and, after repeating it once or twice, then the other. A similar series, starting at the centre and moving laterally, should then be applied over the anterior aspect of the pubic bone. Great care should be taken not to use undue pressure as the area is sensitive at the best of times and may be acutely so if there is dysfunction associated with the insertions into these structures. A series of deep slow movements is then performed, via the

thumb, along the superior and inferior aspects of the inguinal ligament, starting at the pubic bone and running up to and beyond the iliac crest.

The thumbs or fingertips may then be insinuated beneath the lateral rectus border at its lower margins, and deep pressure applied towards the midline. The hand or thumb should then slowly move cephalid in short stages whilst maintaining this medial pressure. This lifts the connective tissue from its underlying attachments and helps to normalise localised contractures and fibrous infiltrations.

Umbilicus

A series of strokes should then be applied around the umbilicus. Using thumb or flexed fingertips a number of movements of a stretching nature should be performed in which the non-treating hand stabilises the tissue at the start of the stroke which firstly runs from approximately 1 inch superior and lateral to the umbilicus on the right side to the same level on the left side. The non-treating hand then stabilises the tissues at this end-point of the stroke and a further stretching and probing stroke is applied inferiorly to a point about 1 inch inferior and lateral to the umbilicus on the left side. This area is then stabilised and the stroke is applied to a similar point on the right.

The circle is completed by a further stroke upwards, to end at the point at which the series began. This series of movements should have a rhythmical pattern so that as the treating hand reaches the end of its stroke the non-treating hand comes to that point and replaces the contact as a stabilising pressure whilst the treating hand begins its next movement. A series of three or four such circuits of the umbilicus is performed.

Additional strokes may be applied along the midline and the sheaths of the recti muscles from the costal margins downwards.

A soothing culmination to the foregoing 10 to 15 minutes may be applied by a circular clockwise series of movements in which the palm of one hand and the heel of the other alternately circle the whole abdominal area. Thus, with the operator standing to the right of the patient, the palm and fingers of the left hand stroke deeply but gently down the left abdominal structures and then across the lower abdomen towards the operator where, using the heel and palm, the right hand takes over the stroke and proceeds up the right side to the costal margin. At this point it changes direction to run across the upper abdomen where the left hand takes over to repeat this pattern several times.

Specific release techniques may be applied during or after this general treatment. Such abdominal treatment can be repeated several times weekly if indicated but normally once a week is adequate until normality is achieved. In chronic conditions of abdominal or pelvic dysfunction, the NMT approach as described, together with specific release movements and appropriate spinal treatment, will have a profound effect on function in the area.

With an improvement in circulation and drainage and a reduction in tensions, contractions and reflex activities, homeostatic mechanisms are bound to be enhanced.

REFERENCES

Baldry P 1993 Acupuncture, trigger points and musculoskeletal pain. Churchill Livingstone, Edinburgh
Chaitow L 1965 An introduction to Chapman's reflexes. British Journal of Naturopathy
Fielder, Pyott 1955 The science and art of manipulative surgery. American Institute of Manipulative Surgery
Gutstein R 1944 The role of abdominal fibrositis in functional indigestion. Mississippi Valley Medical Journal 66–114
Hoyt H 1953 Segmental nerve lesions as a cause of trigonitis syndrome. Stanford Medical Bulletin 11: 61–64
Jones L 1981 Strain and counterstrain. Academy of Applied Osteopathy, Colorado Springs

Mackenzie J 1909 Symptoms and their interpretation. London
Melnick J 1954 Treatment of trigger mechanisms in gastrointestinal disease. New York State Journal of Medicine 54: 1324–1330
Ranger I et al 1971 Abdominal wall pain due to nerve entrapment. Practitioner 206: 791–792
Theobald G 1949 Relief and prevention of referred pain. Journal of Obstetrics and Gynaecology of British Commonwealth 56: 447–460
Travell J, Simons D 1983 Myofascial pain and dysfunction – trigger point manual. Williams and Wilkins, Baltimore

8

Associated techniques

SOFT TISSUE APPROACHES

In Chapter 6 a detailed description was given of NMT in spinal, cervical, pelvic and intercostal structures, and abdominal techniques were described in Chapter 7. In this chapter a number of additional soft tissue approaches which are frequently employed alongside NMT (listed in Box 8.1) will be outlined in alphabetical rather than any other sequence.

Elbow technique

In treating certain muscle groups, notably the gluteals and the sacrospinalis group, it is

---

Box 8.1   Additional soft tissue approaches

- Elbow technique
- Chill-and-stretch technique
- Deep tissue technique
- Induration technique
- Integrated neuromuscular inhibition technique (INIT)
- Ischaemic compression
- Muscle energy techniques
- Percussion technique
- Piriformis technique
- Proprioceptive adjustment
- Psoas technique
- Pump techniques (liver, lymphatics, spleen)
- Skin techniques
- S-contact technique
- Soft tissue manipulation (including massage)
- Special (abdominal) release technique
- Strain/counterstrain
- Tensor fascia lata technique
- Trigger point treatment methods.

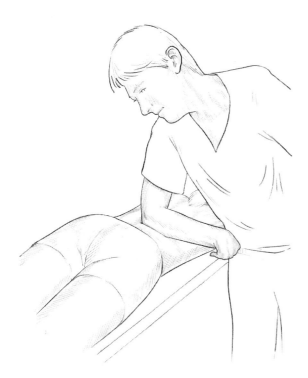

Figure 8.1 Elbow technique applied to paraspinal musculature (see also p. 166).

sometimes difficult, or even impossible, to impart adequate force via the thumb, due to the degree of resistance in the tissues involved. Elbow technique treatment should not be given at the same time as NMT but should be preparatory to it, on a number of occasions, so that NMT can subsequently be effectively applied.

In treating sacrospinalis, for example, the entire spine should be lubricated and the operator should stand on the patient's left side (patient supine, pillow under thorax) (Fig. 8.1).

The right elbow tip is placed just superior to the sacral base, with the forearm at right angles to the patient's body. By flexing the knees slightly and allowing weight to be transferred via the elbow, the operator can apply controlled pressure to the muscles. The elbow is allowed to glide slowly cephalid. If pain is reported, pressure is lessened. Several glides or strokes along the full length of the spine will greatly relax even marked contractions. Similar techniques can be applied to the gluteal area.

Chill-and-stretch technique, trigger point technique

Chilling and stretching a muscle housing a trigger point rapidly assists in deactivation of the abnormal neurological behaviour of the site. Travell and Mennell have described these effects in detail (Mennell 1974, Travell 1952).

Recently, Travell and Simons (1992) have disavowed the use of the vapocoolant approach to the chilling of the area due to environmental considerations relating to ozone depletion. They have instead urged the use of ice massage to achieve the same ends. Whichever approach is used the objective remains the same – to chill the surface tissues while the underlying muscle housing the trigger is stretched (the muscle must not become chilled).

A container of vapocoolant spray with a calibrated nozzle which delivers a moderately fine jet stream, or a source of ice, is needed. The jet stream should have sufficient force to carry in the air for at least 3 feet. A mist-like spray is less desirable. Ice can consist of a cylinder of ice formed by freezing water in a paper cup and then peeling this off the ice. A wooden handle will have been frozen into the ice to allow for its ease of application, as it is rolled from the trigger towards the referred area in a series of sweeps.

The author has found that a cold drink can which has been partially filled with water and then frozen is more suitable since ice applied directly onto skin will rapidly melt and, as Travell has pointed out, the skin must remain dry for this method to be successful because dampness slows the rate of cooling of the skin and may also delay rewarming. An ice-cold metal container, however, can be rolled over the skin and will retain its chilling potential for long enough to achieve the ends desired.

Whichever method is chosen, the patient should be comfortably supported to promote muscular relaxation. If a spray is used the container is held about 2 feet away, in such a manner that the jet stream meets the body surface at an acute angle or at a tangent, not perpendicularly (Fig. 8.2). This lessens the shock of the impact. For the same reason, the stream is sometimes started in

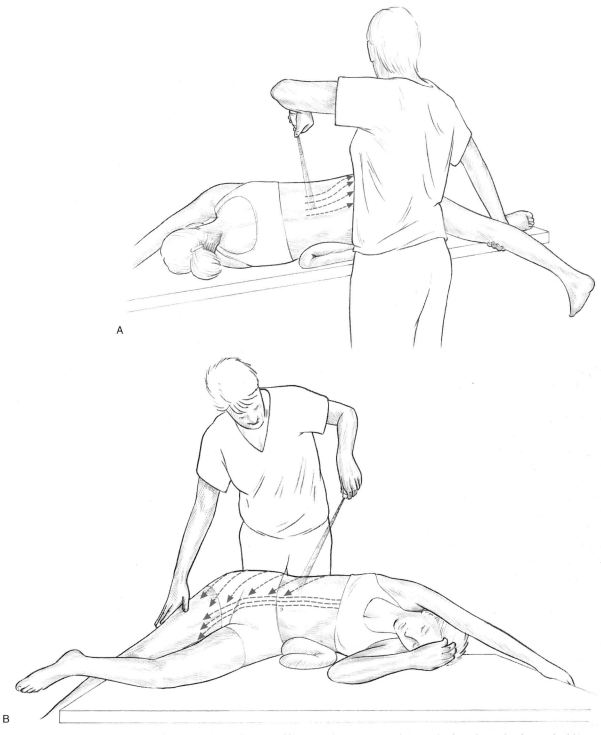

Figure 8.2A,B   Anterior and posterior view of application of vapo-coolant spray to trigger point (quadratus lumborum in this illustration). Muscles housing trigger points are placed at stretch, while a coolant spray is utilised to chill the point and the area between it and the target reference area.

air or on the operator's hand and is gradually brought into contact with the skin overlying the trigger point.

The stream/ice-massage/frozen canister is applied in one direction, not back and forth. Each sweep is started at the trigger point and is moved slowly and evenly outward over the reference zone. Probably it is advantageous to spray or ice-chill both trigger and reference areas, since secondary trigger points are likely to have developed within reference zones when pain is very strong. (The direction of movement is also in line with the muscle fibres towards their insertion.)

The optimum speed of movement of the sweep/roll over the skin seems to be about 4 inches (10 cm) per second. These are repeated in a rhythm of a few seconds on and a few seconds off, until all of the skin over trigger and reference areas has been covered once or twice. If aching or 'cold pain' develops, or if the application of the spray/ice/canister sets off a reference of pain, the interval between applications is lengthened. Care is taken not to frost or blanch the skin.

During the applications of cold, appropriate passive assisted motion should be employed to stretch gently the muscle containing the trigger point. Steady, gentle stretching is usually essential if a satisfactory result is to be achieved. As relaxation occurs, continued stretch should be maintained and after each series of cold applications active motion is tested. The patient is asked to move in the directions which were restricted before spraying was begun. An attempt should be made to restore the full range of motion, but always within the limits of pain, since sudden over-stretching increases existing muscle spasm. At the same time, precautions are taken not to strain the muscles under treatment, either then or during the next few days.

The treatment is continued in this manner until the trigger points (several are usually present) and their respective pain reference zones have been sprayed. The entire procedure may occupy 15 or 20 minutes, and cannot be carried out properly if rushed. However, after chilling the first trigger point for a minute or two and testing it for changes in sensitivity to pressure, one can usually predict whether a successful result will be obtained with the technique. Simple exercises

which utilise the principle of passive stretch should be outlined to the patient, to be carried out several times daily, after the application of gentle heat (hot packs etc.).

The importance of re-establishing normal motion in conjunction with the use of the chilling is well founded. It may be that the brief interruption of pain impulses is insufficient and that input of normal impulses must also occur for the obliteration of trigger points to be successfully achieved.

Deep tissue release technique

In using NMT it is often helpful to apply a local 'tissue release' technique to areas of marked contraction or spasticity. In areas overlying bone the techniques suitable for use in the abdominal region are not applicable. The method recommended is as follows:

The contact on the tissues involved is made by extending the digits of either hand and making firm contact with the area between the first and second metacarpophalangeal joints, taking out the slack of the tissues and engaging a resistance barrier. This contact is rotated clockwise or anti-clockwise in order to increase the tension in the underlying tissues, until the tissues with the greatest resistance are noted and combined barrier is engaged – downwards in a torsional manner. The other hand is then placed over the contact hand so that the downward pressure and rotation are reinforced. In addition, a further direction of stretch should be introduced by the second hand – towards the direction laterally/medially or superiorly/inferiorly, which offers the greatest resistance. The tissues are therefore receiving a direct downward pressure, a rotational stretch and a further degree of stretch in another direction, all maintained by the two treating hands.

The overlying hand should have been placed in such a way that the radial border of the metacarpal base of the thumb is directly over the contact point of the first hand's contact (i.e. over the second metacarpal joint area). The fingers of the overlying hand should be tightly in contact with the lateral border of the contact hand. The final application of the release technique may be performed in one of two ways:

1. The overlying hand executes a short sharp squeeze by flexing the middle finger against the metacarpals of the contact hand. The resulting pressure in the intermetacarpal area provides the 'thrust' or release force. The line of force of this squeeze is towards the operator.

2. The second method of release, which is more suitable for deeper contractions of tissue, is applied via short sharp thrust by the overlying hand against the contact hand, with a simultaneous medial rotation of the contact hand. The line of force in this technique is away from the operator.

This soft tissue approach which emerged from American naprapathy (a form of soft tissue manipulation popular primarily in Sweden and the Chicago area of the USA) and an adhesion releasing method known as 'bloodless surgery', between the two World Wars, has been adapted for use in the UK by McTimoney chiropractic practitioners.

Induration technique (Fig. 8.3)
(Marsh 1969)

Since many patients are too frail or too ill to allow the full NMT treatment to be applied, a useful technique exists to aid in normalising reflex and local areas of the paraspinal musculature. Stoddard (1969) has pointed out that protective

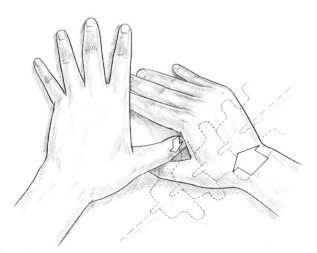

Figure 8.3 Induration technique hand positions. Pressure used on the spinous process is measured in ounces (grams) at most.

spasm in muscle can often indicate underlying pathology (osteoporosis etc.) and clearly deep pressure techniques would be contraindicated in such conditions.

With the patient sitting or lying, the operator, using a very light 'skin–skin' contact which evaluates 'drag' or hills/valleys (see Chapter 5, p. 57), runs the fingertips longitudinally down the side of the spine (side of spine opposite that on which operator is standing) over the transverse processes. Any spot or area of hardened or indurated tissue that also palpates as tender to the patient is marked for attention. Treatment is applied by palpating the sensitive area with the tip of the thumb of one hand whilst applying light pressure towards the painful spot with the soft thenar or hyperthenar eminence of the other hand, which is resting on the spinous process of the vertebra alongside the indurated tissue. Direct pressure (extremely light – ounces only) towards the pain should lessen the degree of tissue contraction and the sensitivity.

If it does not do so then the angle of push on the spinous process towards the painful spot should be varied slightly so that, somewhere within an arc embracing a half circle, an angle of push towards the pain will be found to abolish the pain totally and will lessen the objective feeling of tension. The 'position of ease' is held for around 20 seconds before moving on to the next sensitive area. This technique, which has strong echoes of 'strain/counterstrain' (p. 131) can be used with NMT or instead of the deeper probing measures which, for practical reasons, may be contraindicated (for example, if the patient's condition precluded it due to extreme sensitivity or pathology).

Ischaemic compression

Direct inhibitory pressure has a long history of use in many forms of bodywork including osteopathy in order to achieve a release of hypertonically tense tissues, spasm, cramp etc. Travell (Travell & Simons 1983, 1992) suggests that trigger points receive ischaemic compression ('sustained digital pressure') for a period of between 20 seconds and a minute. The pressure is gradually increased as the trigger point's sensitivity (referred sensation as well as the local discomfort) reduces and the tension of the tissues housing the trigger ('taut band') eases. Stretching techniques should be applied following the compression (see INIT below). The mechanisms involved as seen from a Western perspective would include 'neurological overload', the release of endogenous morphine-like products (endorphins, enkephalins) as well as 'flushing' of tissues with fresh oxygenated blood following the compression. Oriental interpretations would include modulation of energy transmission.

CAUTION: avoid blood vessels and nerves when applying this pressure.

Integrated neuromuscular inhibition technique (INIT) (see Fig. 8.4 and Chapter 9)

This approach involves application of a sequence involving inhibitory (ischaemic) pressure, placement of the tissues into a position of ease to induce a muscle spindle release of excessive tone (see 'positional release' below, p. 131), followed by an introduction by the patient of an isometric contraction of the precise tissues housing the trigger point and finalised by a stretching of the tissues during, or subsequent to, the isometric contraction (see MET below) (Chaitow 1994).

This approach achieves a triple effect – inhibition/ischaemic compression, positional release followed by an isometrically enhanced stretch. The sequence represents a significant advance in deactivating trigger points and the tissues which house them. The initial pressure application (and subsequent positional release and MET) can follow on from the identification of the trigger point during NMT evaluation.

Muscle energy techniques (MET) – including isolytic stretch

Thanks to the influence on their work by Karel Lewit (1992) the more recent edition of Travell and Simons (1992) classic books dealing with myofascial trigger points advocate the use of variations on the theme of muscle energy techniques (MET).

The terms used in MET require clear definition and emphasis:

• An isometric contraction is one in which a muscle, or group of muscles, or a joint, or region of the body, is called upon to contract, or move in a particular direction, and in which that effort is matched by the operator's effort, so that no movement is allowed to take place.

• An isotonic contraction is one in which movement does take place, in that the counterforce offered by the operator is either less than that of the patient, or is greater.

In the first example there would be an approximation of the origin and insertion of the muscle(s) involved, as the effort exerted by the patient more than matches that of the operator. This has a tonic effect on the muscle(s) and is called a concentric isotonic contraction. This method is useful in toning weakened musculature.

Should the second isotonic alternative be employed, the origin and insertion of the muscles involved would not approximate, but would in fact get further apart, due to the greater effort of the operator's counterforce overcoming the muscular effort. This is described as an eccentric isotonic contraction and is also called, in some works, an isolytic contraction. This manoeuvre is useful in cases where there is present, in the soft tissues, a degree of fibrotic change. The effect is to stretch and alter these tissues, thus allowing an improvement in elasticity and circulation.

To achieve an isolytic contraction (eccentric isotonic) the patient should be instructed to use no more than 20% of possible strength on the first contraction, which is resisted and overcome by the operator, in a contraction lasting 7 to 10 seconds. This is then repeated, but with an increased degree of effort on the part of the patient (assuming the first effort was relatively painless). This continuing increase in the amount of force employed in the contracting musculature may be continued until, hopefully, a fairly strong but painless contraction effort is possible, again to be resisted and overcome by the operator. In some muscles, of course, this may

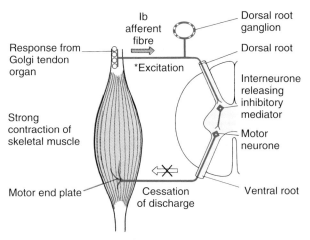

Figure 8.4A Schematic representation of the neurological effects of the loading of the Golgi tendon organs of a skeletal muscle by means of an isometric contraction, which produces a postisometric relaxation effect in that muscle.

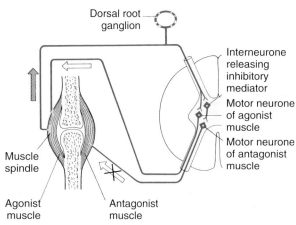

Figure 8.4B Schematic representation of the reciprocal effect of an isometric contraction of a skeletal muscle, resulting in an inhibitory influence on its antagonist.

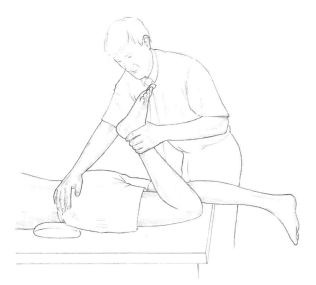

Figure 8.4C MET treatment of left rectus femoris muscle. Note the operator's right hand stabilises the sacrum and pelvis to prevent undue spinal stress during the stretching phase of the treatment.

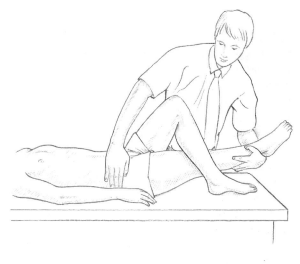

Figure 8.4D MET treatment of TFL. If a standard MET method is being used, the stretch will follow the isometric contraction in which the patient will attempt to move the right leg to the right against sustained resistance. It is important for the operator to maintain stability of the pelvis during the procedure.

require an heroic degree of effort on the part of the operator, and alternative methods would need to be found. NMT would seem to offer one such alternative. The isolytic manoeuvre should have as its ultimate aim a fully relaxed muscle, able to reach its normal resting length. This will not always be possible in one treatment session.

Lewit makes great claims for those aspects of MET (physiological use of patient-generated isometric and isotonic contractions) which are related to achievement of postisometric relaxation and/or reciprocal inhibition.

He says:

By involving muscular physiology we have increasingly engaged the patient's own activity; originally passive manipulative techniques became semi-active, until finally the patient began to learn self-treatment, independent of the therapist. Since these techniques are very effective in producing muscular relaxation, they can also be used to treat muscular spasm, trigger points and even referred pain.

Percussion technique or spondylotherapy

Trigger points can effectively be treated using a series of percussive strokes according to Janet Travell (Travell & Simons 1992).

She states:

The muscle is lengthened to the point of onset of passive resistance. The clinician or patient uses a hard rubber mallet or reflex hammer to hit the trigger point at precisely the same place approximately 10 times. This should be done at a slow rate of no more than one impact per second but, at least, one impact every 5 seconds; the slower rates are likely to be more effective.

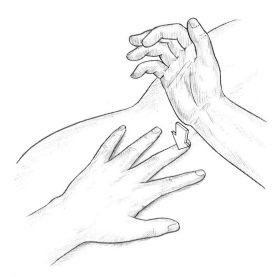

Figure 8.5 Percussion technique (spondylotherapy) for reflexive effects or treatment of trigger points (slow percussion).

She suggests that this enhances or substitutes for intermittent cold with stretch methods as described above (p. 110).

The muscles which she lists as benefiting most include quadratus lumborum (self-applied), brachioradialis, long finger extensors and peroneus longus and brevis. She specifically suggests that anterior and posterior compartment leg muscle should not be treated this way due to the risk of compartment syndrome should bleeding occur in the muscle.

Other uses for percussion

In order to stimulate organs via the spinal pathways, direct percussion techniques have long been employed by osteopathic and chiropractic practitioners. In recent years, Chinese methods involving percussion have dramatically added to our knowledge of the potential of these methods (Zhao-Pu 1991).

Over the past century in the USA a number of mechanical methods of percussion evolved (Abrams 1922), as did effective manual systems in which the middle finger is placed on the appropriate spinous process and the other hand concusses this with a series of rapidly rebounding blows for approximately 5 seconds (Johnson 1939) (Fig. 8.5). During this period, about 15 percussive blows should be applied. This technique is usually applied to a series of three or four (or more) adjacent vertebrae. An example of this is the treatment as above, of the fifth thoracic spinous process, proceeding downwards to the ninth, in the case of liver dysfunction. Treatment would only be applied if the area was painful to palpating pressure. Similarly concussion over tenth, eleventh and twelfth thoracic spinous processes would stimulate kidney function.

A mild 'flare up' of symptoms and increased sensitivity in the area treated would normally indicate that the desired degree of stimulation had been achieved. This form of manual spondylotherapy fits into NMT by virtue of its reflex effects and its easy application. Needless to say, a sound knowledge of spinal mechanics and neurological connections is a prerequisite of such a manoeuvre.

Zhao-pu (1991) describes the Oriental variation on this approach:

Percussion is an important and fundamental manipulation of acupressure therapy, and depending upon the manoeuvre to be carried out is divided into three types – one finger percussion; three finger percussion and five finger percussion. Percussion is also divided into three types according to the degree of force applied.

These three types can be summarised as:

- Light – involving a hand/wrist movement only
- Medium – involving a fixed or semifixed wrist and movement from the elbow
- Strong – which uses force from the shoulder, the whole upper arm being involved with the wrist fixed.

Treatment is offered daily, alternate days or once in 3 days and a course would involve 20 sessions. Patients often receive three courses or more.

Contraindications are acute disease, severe heart disease, TB, malignant tumours, haemorrhagic disease, severe skin disease and poor constitutional states such as malnutrition or asthenia.

Professor Wang Zhao-Pu (whose work using this approach was based on his extensive experience as an orthopaedic surgeon) describes remarkable clinical results involving patients with paralysis and cerebral birth injuries. He states:

Research was carried out on the cerebral haemodynamics of patients with cerebral birth injury before and after acupressure (percussion and pressure techniques) therapy. Scanning techniques were used in monitoring the short half-life radioactive materials through the cerebral circulation; in almost one-third of the patients the regional cerebral blood flow was increased after acupressure therapy ranging from 28 to 60 sessions.

In an introduction to Zhao-Pu's book, Graeme Schofield states:

After cerebral birth injury, significant though the damage may be, there are large areas of the brain and many millions of nerve cells which are still intact.

These areas and the cells they contain are the targets of education for future living.

This approach is therefore not one which produces instant results, but which influences and gradually harnesses the potential for recovery and improvement which is latent in the tissues of the patient. For more information on Oriental bodywork approaches a complete manual of Chinese therapeutic massage (with many aspects which echo NMT methodology) edited by Sun Chengnan is highly recommended (Chengnan 1990).

Piriformis muscle technique
(Retzlaff et al 1974)

The piriformis muscle syndrome results from contracture of the muscle either due to trauma or repetitive mechanical or postural stress. The effects of piriformis shortening can be circulatory, neurological and functional, inducing pain and paraesthesia of the affected limb as well as alterations to pelvic and lumbar function since the muscle anchors the sacrum to the femur. Diagnosis usually hinges on the absence of spinal causative factors for the symptoms.

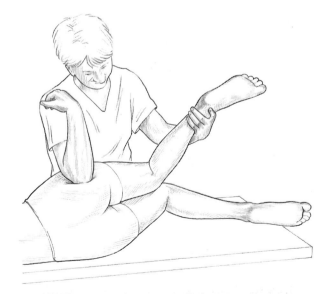

Figure 8.6 Combined ischaemic compression (elbow or thumb) and MET applied to piriformis muscle.

Piriformis muscle syndrome is frequently characterised by such bizarre symptoms that they may seem unrelated. One characteristic complaint is a persistent, severe, radiating low-back pain extending from the sacrum to the hip joint, over the gluteal region and the posterior portion of the upper leg and down to the popliteal space. In the most severe cases the patient will be unable to lie or stand comfortably, and changes in position will not relieve the pain. Intense pain will occur when the patient sits or squats.

A common sign of the piriformis syndrome is a persistent external rotation of the upper leg. This indication, which is known as the positive piriformis sign, is easily detected when the patient is examined in the supine position.

The buttock on the same side as the piriformis lesion is usually sensitive to touch or palpation. Severe pain may occur when pressure is applied to the area over the piriformis muscle and its tendinous insertion on the head of the greater trochanter.

Another diagnostic sign may be the shortening of the leg on the affected side due to contracture of the piriformis muscle. In cases where the leg on the opposite side appears shortened, it is probable that some other dysfunction exists and that the condition is not directly related to the piriformis syndrome.

The patient may also mention pain that follows the distribution pattern of the sciatic nerve to the level of the popliteal space and sometimes to the more distal branches of this nerve. When the common perineal nerve is involved, there may be a paraesthesia of the posterior surface of the upper leg and some portions of the lower leg.

One of the most perplexing problems arising from the piriformis syndrome is the involvement of the pudendal nerve and blood vessels. This nerve with its branches, provides the major sensory innervation of the perineal skin and the somatic motor innervation of much of the external genitalia and related perineal musculature in both women and men. The pudendal blood vessels supply essentially the same areas. The pudendal nerve, after passing through the greater sciatic foramen, re-enters the pelvis by way of the lesser sciatic foramen. In a significant percentage of people the perineal and tibial components of the sciatic nerve actually pass through the piriformis muscle giving rise in these individuals to a greater likelihood of severe symptoms if the muscle shortens or is stressed (Polstein 1991). Compression of the pudendal nerve and blood vessels can result in serious problems involving the functioning of the genitalia in both sexes. Since external rotation of the upper legs is required for women during coitus, if there were interference with the blood supply and innervation of the genitalia, it is understandable that a female patient might complain of pain during sexual intercourse. This could also be a basis for impotency in men.

Ischaemic compression applied by thumb or elbow, with or without MET, is usually sufficient to remedy the problem.

Piriformis treatment

Method (a). Patient lying on side, affected side uppermost, legs flexed at hip and knees. The operator's elbow is applied to the piriformis tendon and heavy downward pressure is exerted for 10 seconds at a time, up to ten times, with a few seconds rest in between. This should relieve symptoms of a traumatic nature where the condition is not of too long standing and where no spinal or sacroiliac involvement is present. (See Fig. 8.6.)

Method (b). In an alternative approach to piriformis contracture the patient lies on the non-affected side with the knees flexed and the upper legs perpendicular to the body. The operator places an elbow on the piriformis musculo-tendinous junction and a steady pressure of 20–30 lbs (9–13 kg) is applied. With the other hand, the foot is abducted so that it will force an internal rotation of the upper leg. The leg is held in the rotated position for periods of up to 2 minutes. A periodic introduction of an isometric contraction against operator resistance (patient lightly applies force to externally rotate hip, contracting piriformis) for up to 10 seconds at a time will allow for increased range of rotation following the contraction.

This procedure is repeated two or three times. The patient is then placed in the supine position and the affected leg is tested for freedom of both external and internal rotation.

Proprioceptive adjustment (applied kinesiology) (Figs 8.7 & 8.8)
(Walther 1988)

Kinesiological muscle tone correction utilises two key receptors in muscles to achieve its effects. A muscle in spasm may be helped to relax by the application of direct pressure (using approximately 2 lbs of pressure) away from the belly of the muscle, in the area of the Golgi tendon organs, and/or by the application of the same amount of pressure towards the belly of

STRENGTHEN

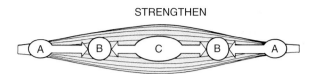

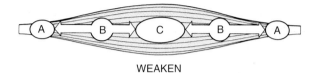

WEAKEN

A = golgi tendon organs

B = belly of muscle

C = muscle spindle

Figure 8.7 Proprioceptive manipulation of muscles (see text).

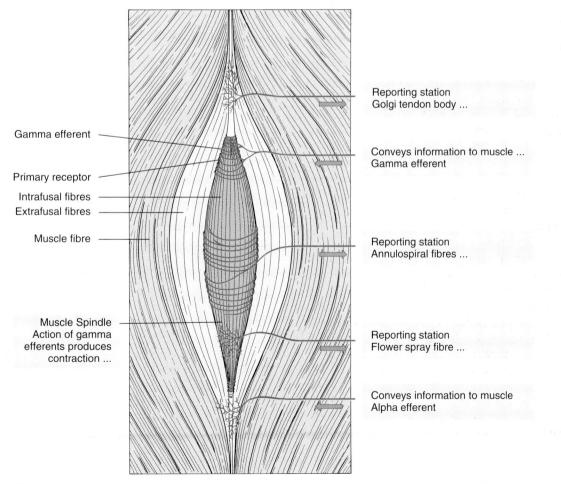

Gamma efferent

Primary receptor

Intrafusal fibres

Extrafusal fibres

Muscle fibre

Muscle Spindle
Action of gamma
efferents produces
contraction ...

Reporting station
Golgi tendon body ...

Conveys information to muscle ...
Gamma efferent

Reporting station
Annulospiral fibres ...

Reporting station
Flower spray fibre ...

Conveys information to muscle
Alpha efferent

Figure 8.8 Illustration of muscle spindles, showing Golgi tendon organ and neural pathways to and from these reporting stations.

the muscle, in the area of the muscle spindle cells.

The precise opposite effects (i.e. toning or strengthening the muscle) are said to be achieved by applying pressure away from the belly of the muscle, in the muscle spindle region, and towards the belly of the muscle in the tendon organ region.

Note that Janda (1990, 1992) in particular takes the view, that weakness in a muscle can best be addressed by dealing with (stretching etc.) hypertonicity in its antagonist(s).

Psoas technique

In postural distortion such as scoliotic or marked lumbar lordotic conditions as well as in many acute low back and sciatic cases, the iliopsoas muscle is found to be involved.

Test for psoas contraction

X-ray diagnosis is the only sure method of determining psoas contraction and its effects on spinal function. A simple test involves patient lying at end of bed with unaffected (non-tested) side leg in full flexion and tested leg hanging freely in space. If the thigh is parallel with the floor/table psoas is considered not to be shortened; however, if it is elevated shortness is presumed.

Psoas technique – direct inhibitory pressure

Method (a). Patient lies on back with knees flexed, hands at side. Practitioner stands on side opposite contracted psoas. One hand presses down firmly through the linea alba, 3 to 4 inches (7–10 cm) below the umbilicus, until the probing fingers contact the body of the fourth to fifth lumbars. The practitioner then gently slides fingers laterally, until the body of the psoas is felt, and maintains firm but gentle pressure for about a minute (Fig. 8.9A,B).

Method (b). Same as (a) except practitioner is seated on opposite side to contraction. Same contact with fingers through linea alba but with the other hand bringing the flexed leg towards the opposite shoulder and rotating the pelvis against probing fingers.

Method (c). Same as (a) except the practitioner places his flexed leg on the table to support the patient's leg on contracted psoas side. In this manner, both hands are free to support each other as they penetrate heavier abdomens (Fig. 8.9C).

Method (d). Same as (a) except practitioner's flexed leg supports both of patient's legs. This is especially useful when there exists a contraction of both psoas muscles (Fig. 8.9D).

A number of MET and SCS approaches also exist for safely treating psoas and appropriate texts should be consulted for details of these.

Pump techniques – lymphatics, liver or spleen
(Fielding 1983)

Lymphatic pump method (a). Patient is prone, pillow under chest, arms over the side, operator standing at the head of the table, facing caudad. The operator's thumbs are pressed, bilaterally onto the intertransverse spaces, starting at the base of the neck. Pressure is exerted towards the floor as the patient swings the arms forwards. This swing is repeated each time the thumbs move down one intervertebral space. This will have a stimulating effect on the lymphatic drainage of the body as a whole. The effect is enhanced if the patient inhales deeply during the procedure and coincides the strong swing of the arms with the cycle of the breath (see Fig. 8.10A)

Lymphatic pump method (b). (Sleszynski et al 1993) The patient lies supine, knees and hips flexed. The operator is at the head of the table with hands spread across the patient's chest, below the clavicles, with thumbs resting next to each other on the sternum, fingers spread laterally. Pressure is introduced by the operator, in a downwards and caudad direction, which is just sufficient to overcome resistance. The patient continues to breathe normally, and does not resist the repetitive pressure of the operator, which should be between a rate which corresponds with the respiratory rate, and 150 per

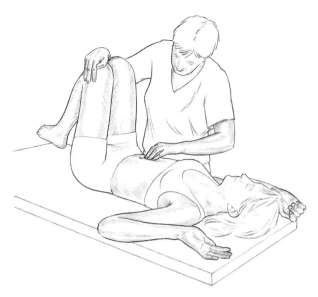

Figure 8.9A Direct finger pressure applied to right side of psoas attachment to anterior spinal structures.

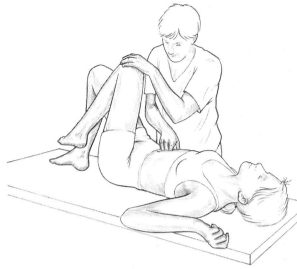

Figure 8.9B Use of altered knee positions to enhance access to psoas attachments.

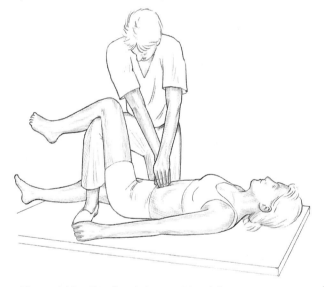

Figure 8.9C Two-handed contact to reinforce psoas contact, with use of operator's leg to support patient's contralateral leg in order to modify overlying muscle and psoas tension.

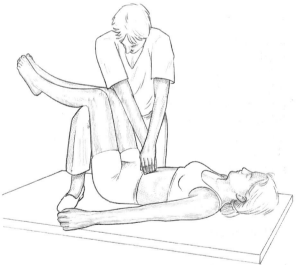

Figure 8.9D Both patient's legs supported by operator's leg as a means of modifying psoas tension in cases of bilateral psoas dysfunction.

Figure 8.9 Psoas techniques.

minute. The patient breathes through the mouth, and the pumping action takes over the respiratory function (see Fig. 8.10B). This should continue for at least 3 minutes and up to 5 minutes.

In babies, the method can be used with one hand over the sternum, the other under the spine with the baby cradled or seated on the operator's lap. The effect of this is a dramatic improvement in lymphatic drainage. It is useful in all cases of oedema and infection. It also has a

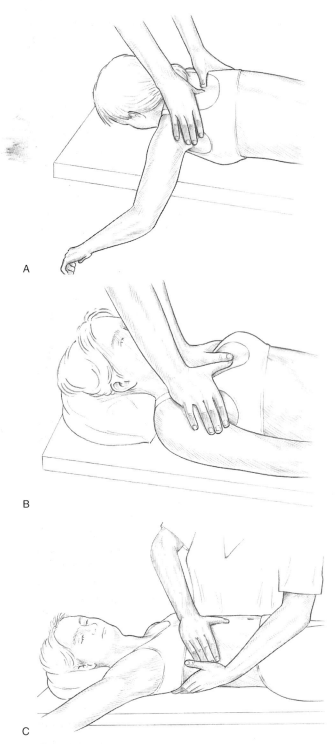

A

B

C

Figure 8.10 Lymphatic pump techniques.
A – Patient prone.   B — Patient supine.   C — Liver pump technique.

beneficial effect on immune function (Hoag 1969).

The use of Chapman's reflexes (see Ch. 4, p. 53) will provide additional localised drainage, which would support the general drainage and stimulation of lymphatic function, which the methods described above, provide. These methods are particularly useful in children. None of the procedures described should be painful.

Liver/spleen pump method. A simple measure, via which function of either the liver or spleen may be enhanced involves the operator standing on the side opposite the organ which is being stimulated (left side of patient, reaching across for the liver, and vice versa for the spleen). Patient is supine, knees and hips flexed. The operator's caudad hand is placed under the lower ribs, and the other is placed anteriorly, just medial to the costal cartilages of the lower five ribs (Fig. 8.10C). Alternative bimanual compression should initially be carried out in a direct anterior-posterior direction. This is done approximately twenty times per minute, for 1 to 2 minutes. After this, the direction of the pumping action should be more in an anterolateral direction, for a further minute. The effect on the spleen is such as to increase the leucocyte count by an average of 2200 cells per cubic millimetre (Castlio 1955).

SKIN TECHNIQUES

Skin rolling (Fig. 8.11) is a useful all-purpose approach which involves the use of either or both hands. The fingers draw tissue towards the operator whilst the ball(s) of the thumb(s) roll over the gathered mound of tissue. In this way the tissue is effectively lifted, stretched and squeezed. The most useful areas of application occur where the tissues lie tight to the underlying structures, such as directly over the shoulder joint and on the lateral aspect of the thigh. The squeezing pressure imparted by the roll of the thumb can be extremely uncomfortable and care should be exercised during its application. The angle of stretch, pull and roll may be varied and repeated several times to impart maximum stimulus to the reflex effects

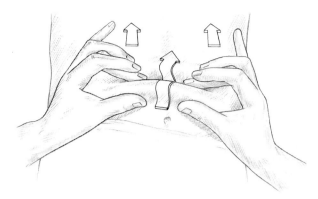

Figure 8.11 Skin rolling method.

and to stimulate circulation and drainage. Stanley Lief and Boris Chaitow employed this simple, yet effective manoeuvre as part of their general treatment. The latter described its usefulness as follows (Chaitow 1983):

One of my favourite techniques to enhance nerve and blood circulation is 'skin rolling'. Between the skin and the muscular and bony structures it covers, is a veritable network of blood and nerve structures and functions which can, and often do, fail to achieve their full, effective circulation for high efficiency and health because the skin is often so adhered to its lower structures (fascia) that circulation and function is appreciably reduced. This of course adversely affects the efficiency and health of the patient. There is probably no formula that will enhance this aspect of function more effectively than 'skin rolling'. A specific example of its effective benefit is to skin-roll a major joint such as a shoulder in conditions of articular rheumatism, arthritis, neuritis, frozen shoulder etc.

Treating hyperalgesic skin zones – stretching

As noted in earlier chapters, the skin overlying regions, or points of reflex activity, will frequently be found to have markedly reduced elasticity, and to adhere to underlying structures. Assessment of these areas is described in Chapter 5 (p. 72).

To treat a local area of hyperalgesia the fingertips, or the ulnar aspects of the crossed hands, are placed together on the affected skin surface and the tissues are stretched apart, to their easy resistance barrier, as the fingers, or hands, separate. In order to establish the presence or lack of physiological elasticity, the skin is stretched in various directions. If restriction is noted then the tissues are held in a painlessly stretched position, until a degree of release is noted. This should take no more than 10 seconds. The same area may be stretched in this manner in various appropriate directions. The release of the tissues is itself the therapeutic effort, providing reflex stimulus. The subsequent maintenance of the free elastic state of the tissues is evidence of an improvement in the causative factors. Naturally, if underlying factors maintain the reflex activity, whether this be musculoskeletal or visceral dysfunction, the improvement will be short lived. HSZ is useful diagnostically and prognostically (Lewit 1992).

Lewit states:

If pain is due to the HSZ, this method is quite as effective as needling, electrostimulation and other similar methods. Moreover, it is entirely painless, and can be applied by the patient himself.

Such zones are frequently noted with musculoskeletal conditions, and in chronic pain syndromes. In cases of recurrent headache, HSZ are found medially below the mastoid process, at the temples and eyebrows, and on the forehead above the eyebrows, and on both sides of the nose. This correlates with many of Bennett's neurovascular reflexes as discussed in previous chapters.

Skin – pinch-roll technique for HSZ. With the patient prone, the operator's hands are placed so that the fingers are more cephalid, and the thumb more caudad. The fingers draw skin towards the thumb, which lifts this fold. The tissue thus held, between the thumb and fingers, is then lifted away from the body, and rolled slightly upwards (towards the fingers cephalid). The degree of stretch and/or pinch employed is a variable factor which the operator may decide upon, depending upon the amount of stimulus called for. Either skin alone, or skin and underlying tissue, may be lifted, stretched and stimulated (pinched) in this way. Traditional Chinese medicine calls for this procedure to be undertaken from the base of the spine upwards, for a tonifying effect, and from the neck downwards, for a sedating effect.

'S' contact technique for tissue release (Fig. 8.12). (Lewit 1992) In order to achieve a relaxation of a specific area of muscle tension the hands should be positioned in such a way as to allow thumb or hand pressure to be applied across the fibres of a contracted or indurated muscle or soft tissue area so that the contacts are travelling in opposite directions to each other. In this way, as pressure is applied simultaneously with each thumb or hand the tissues between the two contacts will progressively have the slack removed and be placed in a slightly stretched situation in which they can be held until release occurs (or 'springing' is introduced). This technique can be applied along the course of particularly spastic and hard unyielding tissues, as well as the basic NMT thumb technique.

It is called 'S' contact because the tissues being treated form that shape as the strokes are performed. The same procedure exactly may be used, but with a flicking action of the thumb to complete the stroke, once effective tension has been created in the tissues by the opposing thumbs. This 'springing' has the effect of stimulating local circulation most effectively and if the tissues are not too sensitive, may be effective in breaking down infiltrated or indurated tissues.

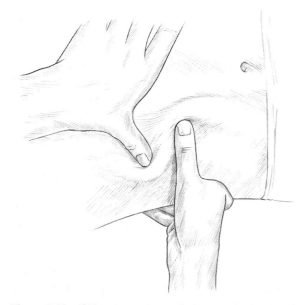

Figure 8.12 'S' bend pressure applied to tense or fibrotic musculature.

SOFT TISSUE MANIPULATION – INCLUDING MASSAGE

The term 'soft tissue manipulation' can be used to encompass all manual methods which address tissues other than bone, and include the main topics of this book. Neuromuscular technique, muscle energy techniques and positional release methods (strain–counterstrain etc.) can (with other modalities such as chilling agents) all be used as effective measures to detect and help to normalise dysfunctional soft tissues, including areas housing noxious trigger points which can themselves be responsible for the promotion or maintenance of muscular weakness, muscular contraction, pain, vasodilatation, vasoconstriction, tissue degeneration, gastrointestinal, respiratory and a myriad other disorders, including emotional and 'psychological' disorders.

The logical approach to correction of dysfunction involving shortened tight musculature, is to lengthen and stretch these tissues. NMT and muscle energy techniques are useful in achieving this. Such an approach may involve any combination of the many variations of these techniques, and could include deep NMT, followed by isometric methods, which employ postisometric relaxation, as well as reciprocal inhibition, and also isotonic (isolytic) methods which contribute towards breaking down fibrotic contractions.

Correct sequence of therapy

Treatment of dysfunction associated with muscles which have become weak could involve initial attention to their antagonists which may be inhibiting them, as well as to isotonic concentric MET methods applied to weak muscles themselves plus exercises specific to the area. General postural and body-toning exercises could follow. Before such exercise is initiated, it is important to discover and treat local dysfunction within shortened or weakened muscles – such as trigger points – and NMT will usefully help towards achieving this. It is often useful to allow the results of normalisation of shortened muscles to unfold without confusing the issue by exercising the weakened antagonists too soon, since a natural toning effect will occur when inhibitory influences are removed. If, after several weeks of treatment of the shortened, contracted, postural muscles and their trigger points, there is not an observable and measurable improvement in the weak antagonists, then MET and exercise could usefully be introduced to these as well.

The use of gentle functional techniques, such as those of Lawrence Jones (strain/counterstrain, for example) are suitable for combining with NMT and MET methods. By using muscle energy techniques to help to lengthen shortened structures, and NMT to aid in this, as well as in identifying localised areas of soft tissue dysfunction (myofascial trigger points or other forms of soft tissue dysfunction) the operator has a wide array of diagnostic and therapeutic methods, literally at his finger tips.

Massage

We should not lose sight of the tried and tested effects of massage on the soft tissues. The degree of that effect will vary with the type of soft tissue manipulation employed, and the nature of the patient and the problem.

Soft tissue techniques, apart from those specifically associated with NMT, may include:

Petrissage. This involves wringing and stretching movements.

These techniques attempt to 'milk' the tissues of waste products, and assist in circulatory interchange. The manipulations press and roll the muscles under the hands. Petrissage may be performed with one hand, where the area requiring treatment is small, or more usually with two hands. In extremely small areas (base of the thumb for example) it can be performed by two fingers, or finger and thumb. It is applicable to skin, fascia, muscle, etc. In a relaxing mode, the rhythm should be around 10 to 15 cycles per minute, and to induce stimulation this can rise to around 35 cycles per minute. It is usually a cross-fibre activity.

Unhurried, deep pressure is the usual mode of application in large muscle masses, which require stretching and relaxing. The thenar eminence or the hyperthenar eminence, are the main strong contacts, but fingers, or the whole of the hand, may be involved. An example of this movement, as applied to the low back, would be as follows:

Method. Both hands are placed on one side of the prone patient, one at the level of the upper gluteals, the other several inches higher, each hand will describe circles, counterclockwise, but they will do so in such a manner that as one hand moves laterally from the spine the other hand will begin to move towards the spine from a point a little higher on the back. The contact can be the flat hand, or the thenar or hyperthenar eminences.

One handed petrissage may involve treatment of an arm for example. In this the hand lifts and squeezes the tissues, making a small circular motion. Many other variations exist in this technique, which is mainly aimed at achieving general relaxation of the muscles, and improved circulation and drainage.

Kneading. This is used to improve fluid exchange and to achieve relaxation of tissues. The hands shape themselves to the contours of the area being treated. The tissues between the hands, as they approximate each other, are lifted and pressed downwards and together. This squeezes and kneads the tissues. Each position receives three or four cycles of this sort before the lower hand takes the place of the upper hand, and it glides upwards to its next position. Little lubricant is required, as the hands should cling to the part being manipulated, lifting it, and pressing and sliding only when changing position. A degree of deep stroking is used to move fluid contents.

Inhibition. This involves application of pressure directly to the belly or origins or insertions of contracted muscles or to local soft tissue dysfunction, for a minute or more, or in a 'make and break' manner, to reduce hypertonic contraction or for reflex effects.

Effleurage. Effleurage (stroking) is used to induce relaxation and reduce fluid congestion – applied superficially or at depth. This is a relaxing drainage technique, which should be used, as appropriate, to initiate or terminate other manipulative methods. Pressure is usually even throughout the strokes, which are applied with the whole hand in contact. Any combination of areas may be thus treated. Superficial tissues are usually rhythmically treated by this method. Since drainage is one of its main aims, peripheral areas are often treated, in order to drain venous or lymphatic fluid towards the centre. Lubricants are usually used.

A useful low back variation is the use of stroking horizontally across the tissues. The operator stands facing the side of the patient, at waist level. The caudad hand rests on the upper gluteals, and the cephalad hand on the area just above the iliac crest. One hand strokes from the side closest to the operator away to the other side, as the other hand applies a pulling stroke, from the far side towards the operator. The two hands pass, and then without changing position, reverse direction and pass each other again. The degree of pressure used is optional, and the technique can be continued in one position for several strokes, before moving the hands upwards on the back.

This is but one of many variations on the theme of stroking; a technique which is relaxing to the patient and useful in achieving fluid alteration.

Vibration and friction. Vibration and friction are used near origins and insertions, and near bony attachments, for relaxing effects on the muscle as a whole. This is used to reach below superficial tissues. It is performed by small circular or vibratory movements, with the tips of fingers or thumb. The heel of the hand may also be used. The aim is to move the tissues under the skin, and not the skin itself. It is applied, for example, to joint spaces, around bony prominences and near well-healed scar tissue to reduce adhesions. Pressure is applied gradually, until the tolerance of the patient is reached. The minute circular or vibratory movement is introduced, and this is maintained for some seconds before gradual release and movement to another position.

Stroking techniques are used subsequently, to drain tissues and to relax the patient.

Stretching. Stretching can be used along or across the belly of muscles using heel of hand, thumb or fingers applied slowly and rhythmically. Cross fibre friction is one such approach which involves pressure across the muscle fibres, and in this form the stroke moves across the skin, in a series of short deep strokes. One thumb following the other, in a series of such strokes, laterally from the spinous processes, aids in reduction of local contraction and fibrous changes. Short strokes along the fibres of muscle may also be used, in which the skin contact is maintained, and the tissues under the skin are moved. This requires deep short strokes, and is useful in areas of fibrous change. Thumbs are the main contact in this variation.

Another variation on the treatment of fibrotic change, is the use of deep friction, which may be applied to muscle, ligament or joint capsule, across the long axis of the fibres, using the thumb or any variation of the finger contacts. The index finger, supported by the middle finger, or the middle finger with its two adjacent fingers supporting it, makes for a strong treatment unit. Precise localisation of target tissues is possible with this sort of contact.

The methods listed above do not represent a comprehensive description of massage-based, soft tissue techniques, but are meant to indicate some of the basic movements available from this source. Some, or all of these are bound to be involved in any attempt to deal with soft tissue problems.

Other methods which we would associate with the above techniques of traditional massage might include the various applications of NMT, as described in this text, as well as connective tissue massage techniques which are used primarily for reflex effects.

Effects explained

How are the various effects of massage and soft tissue manipulation explained? A combination of physical effects occur apart from the undoubted anxiety reducing influences (Sandler 1983) which involve a number of biochemical changes, for example plasma cortisol and catecholamine concentrations alter markedly as anxiety levels drop, and depression is also reduced (Field 1992). Serotonin levels rise as sleep is enhanced – even in severely ill patients, preterm infants, cancer patients and people with irritable bowel problems as well as HIV-positive individuals for example (Acolet 1993, Ferel-Tory 1993, Ironson et al 1993, Weinrich & Weinrich 1990).

On a physical level pressure, as applied in deep kneading or stroking along the length of a muscle, tends to displace its fluid content. Venous, lymphatic and tissue drainage is thereby encouraged. The replacement of this with fresh oxygenated blood aids in normalisation via increased capillary filtration and venous capillary pressure. This reduces oedema and the effects of pain-inducing substances which may be present (Hovind et al 1974, Xujian 1990).

Massage also produces a decrease in the sensitivity of the gamma efferent control of the muscle spindles, and thereby reduces any shortening tendency of the muscles (Puustjarvi et al 1990).

Pressure techniques, such as are used in NMT, and the methods employed in MET, have a direct effect on the Golgi tendon organs, which detect the load applied to the tendon or muscle. These have an inhibitory capability, which can cause the entire muscle to relax.

The Golgi tendon organs are set in series in the muscle, and are affected by both active and passive contraction of the tissues. The effect of any system which applies longitudinal pressure or stretch to the muscle, will be to evoke this reflex relaxation. The degree of stretch has, however, to be great, as there is little response from a small degree of stretch. The effect of MET, articulation techniques, and various functional balance techniques depends to a large extent on these tendon reflexes (Sandler 1983).

We are in the midst of a change in the concepts of manual therapy which has far-reaching implications. One of the major changes is the restoration of the soft tissue component to centre stage, rather than the peripheral role to which it has been assigned in the past as ever more general health problems are found to involve musculoskeletal dysfunction, for example in chronic fatigue conditions (Chaitow 1990).

Lewit (1985) discusses aspects of what he describes as the 'no man's land', which lies between neurology, orthopaedics and rheumatology which, he says, is the home of the vast majority of patients with pain derived from the locomotor system, and in whom no definite pathomorphological changes are found. He makes the suggestion that these be termed cases of 'functional pathology of the locomotor system'. These include most of the patients attending osteopathic, chiropractic and physiotherapy practitioners.

The most frequent symptom of individuals involved in this area of dysfunction is pain, which may be reflected clinically by reflex changes such as muscle spasm, myofascial trigger points, hyperalgesic skin zones, periosteal pain points, or a wide variety of other sensitive areas which have no obvious pathological origin. Since the musculoskeletal system is the largest energy user in the body, it is no surprise that fatigue is a feature of chronic changes in the musculature.

It is a major part of the role of NMT to help in identifying such areas, and also offering some help in differential diagnosis. NMT and other soft tissue methods are then capable of normalising many of the causative aspects of these myriad sources of pain and disability.

Specific (abdominal) release techniques (Fig. 8.13)

Boris Chaitow, who worked closely with Lief wrote (Chaitow 1983):

Stanley Lief taught that manipulation (bony or soft tissue) should not only be confined to the spine itself but also locally to every possible area related to the particular symptom or stress. On the whole the neuromuscular technique he devised is applied with the thumb, as this universally useful digit lends itself to the pattern of pressure and technique required, and is at the same time highly sensitive in diagnostic palpation.

One of the areas of the body which Stanley Lief found uniquely amenable for his soft tissue technique is the abdomen. It can be safely asserted that there is no one in middle age and older who has not, unfortunately, developed some of the tensions, contractions, adhesions, nerve and muscle spasms in various parts of the gastro-intestinal tract and

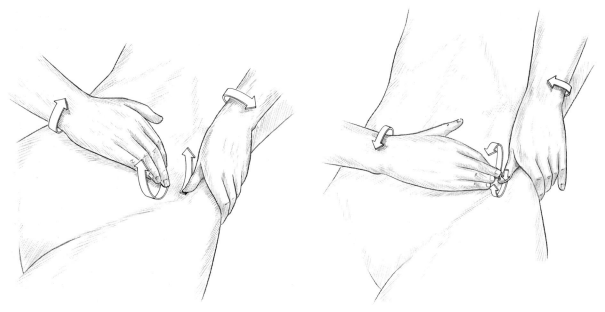

Figure 8.13A Both hands release tissue which has been taken to its elastic barrier in various directions — compressed, stretched apart, counter-rotated, and finally 'sprung'.

Figure 8.13B The right hand springs the restricted tissues, after all slack has been removed and some stretch applied, while the left hand acts mainly to produce a stabilising contact against which a precisely controlled force is applied.

Figure 8.13 Specific release technique as used in treatment of adhesions and tensor fascia lata restrictions.

abdominal cavity so common today. All these would normally be outside the scope of the conventional manipulator. But, with the neuromuscular technique, a practitioner can achieve almost dramatic benefits in local stresses and in health in general. He devised for the abdomen the special technique he called 'bloodless surgery' – a method of breaking up deep-seated adhesions and contractions. It also enables the operator to improve function and circulation related to female problems such as dysmenorrhoea, menorrhagia and amenorrhoea, fibroids etc.

Lief used methods derived from an American system of manipulative or 'bloodless surgery' to amplify his abdominal techniques. His and Boris Chaitow's technique is presented here. These 'release' techniques can be applied to soft areas of the body (e.g. the throat) as well as to the abdomen. The original concept of 'bloodless surgery' was that adhesions were being 'peeled' away from their anchorage by the technique and in some cases this might have been so. However, its current application is to any area of tight, fibrosed, spastic, contracted or adhering soft tissue in the abdominal region or elsewhere – for

example on the lateral thigh in tense and contracted fascial tissues. The most dramatic improvements in function were noted by Lief and Chaitow after its use in such conditions as spastic or atonic constipation, visceroptosis, dysmenorrhoea, menorrhagia etc. as well as ill-defined abdominal congestion and pain. The author confines its use to deeply indurated muscle and fascial structures such as are found in tensor fascia lata (see below in this chapter, p. 132).

Precisely what takes place after abdominal release technique is open to conjecture. An improvement in tone and circulation and usually of general function is the most obvious result. It is a matter of debate whether this is because of a release of a long-held contractive state in the soft tissues or because of an actual breaking of adhesions or because of some other mechanism.

A general abdominal neuromuscular treatment precedes the first specific release technique (Technique A, p. 129). This serves to both relax and tone the area in a general manner whilst enabling the operator to localise areas which feel indurated or contracted objectively, as well as noting all areas of subjective sensitivity as reported by the patient.

It is these (a) tight, contracted and (b) sensitive areas that receive the release technique. The ability of the operator to localise accurately such areas is obviously critical and must be a matter for constant practice until the hands and fingers feel such abnormalities as a matter of course. To this end it is suggested that the middle finger of the right hand (in a right-handed operator) be trained to seek and mark those areas that will require specific release techniques. This requires practising the use of the hand in a position where the fingers are flexed so that the middle finger is slightly more prominent than its neighbours.

This aids its task of palpating specifically the tissues being probed. The non-searching fingers support the hand and are involved in assessing tissue tension as well as holding movable soft tissues as an aid to the palpating finger.

The patient should be supine with knees flexed and feet as close to the buttocks as possible for maximum abdominal relaxation and with the head on a small pillow. The operator should stand facing the patient on the side opposite that being treated, i.e. to treat the left inguinal area the operator stands, knees flexed, leaning across from the patient's right side. This allows the tissues being manipulated to be drawn towards the operator in a controlled manner whereas such a procedure performed with the hands being pushed away from the operator, as would be the case if working from the side being treated, would cause a degree of pushing or gouging of the tissues, resulting in pain and a lack of fine control.

Technique A. Having located an area of contracted (often sensitive) tissue the middle finger locates the point of maximum resistance and the tissues are drawn towards the operator, to the limit of pain-free movement. The middle finger and its neighbours should be flexed, fairly rigid and be imparting force in two directions at this stage, i.e. downwards (towards the floor) and towards the operator. (In 'bloodless surgery' techniques the right hand is always on the 'adhesion' and the other contact on the organ to

which the lesion is attached.) With the fingers maintaining the above position, the thumb of the left hand is placed almost immediately – no more than quarter of an inch (6 mm) away – adjacent to the middle finger of the right hand, in such a way that a downward pressure (towards the floor) will provide a fulcrum point against which force can be applied via the right hand, in order to stretch or reduce the degree of contraction in the tissue (or indeed to break or 'peel' adhesions). The thumb should also be flexed and the contact can be via its tip or its lateral border or a combination of the two.

The idea of a fulcrum is important since the two points of contact are both on soft tissue structures and the effect of the manipulation is achieved, not by pulling or twisting these apart, but by a combination of movements which impart force in several directions at the same time. This is accomplished by a quick clockwise movement of the right hand (middle finger contact) against the stabilising anchorage of the left thumb. Movement of the thumb during this release is not essential or necessary. However, Boris Chaitow does impart a degree of additional torsional force by releasing the thumb contact in an anticlockwise direction at the moment of manipulation.

With both hands in contact, as described, and the contact digits flexed and rigid, the operator should be so positioned that he is leaning over the affected area, knees flexed with the legs separated for stability, elbows flexed and separated to a point of 180° separation. The force that will be present at the point of contact is a downward one, to which is added a slight separation of the hands, which increases the tension on the affected tissues. The manipulative force is imparted by a quick, flicking of the right contact in a clockwise direction whilst maintaining the left thumb contact (or taking it in an anticlockwise direction).

The effect of the right hand movement would be to snap the right elbow towards the operator's side. If a double release is performed then both elbows will come rapidly to the sides. The amount of force imparted should be controlled so that no pain is felt by the patient. The essence of this technique is the speed with which it is applied and its success depends upon this as much as the correct positioning of the hands and the exact location of the area of tissue dysfunction. The same procedure can be repeated several times on the same area and the release of a number of such areas of contracted or indurated tissue, at any one treatment, is usual. The same thumb contact is often maintained whilst variations in the direction of tissue tension are dealt with by slightly altering the angle of the right hand contact and manipulative effort. If, after manipulation, no objective improvement is noted on palpation then the angle of the contacts should be varied. Nothing will be gained, however, by attempting to use excessive force in order to achieve results. Since the degree of soft tissue trauma to the patient is minimal, the after-effects should not include bruising or much discomfort. Any such after-effect would indicate undue pressure or force.

Boris Chaitow describes the above method as follows:

For the technique of NMT on the abdomen referred to already as 'bloodless surgery' palpate with the tips of the fingers of the right hand, and having located the area of abnormal feel, place those four fingers as a group at the distal border of the lesioned area and place the thumb of the left hand along the nails of the right fingers. Give a sharp flick with both hands simultaneously, the left hand thumb being twisted anticlockwise and the fingers of the right hand clockwise (difficult if not impossible to describe on paper). This achieves an appreciable breaking-up, without trauma or hurt to the patient, of tensions, adhesions, congestions etc., both on the wall of the abdomen and structures within the cavity. Obviously these flicks with the hands have to be repeated a number of times to feel a discernible difference in the lesioned tissue. Stanley Lief achieved dramatic changes in tissue structure and functional improvements in many types of abdominal stresses including digestive problems, gall bladder blockage, gall stones, constipation, spastic colon, colic, colitis, uterine fibroids, dysmenorrhoea, menorrhagia, small non-malignant abdominal tumours, postoperative adhesions etc.

Technique B. A second method for the release of tense, contracted, indurated connective and muscular tissue, is sometimes employed. This requires the same positioning of the patient and the operator, as in method A. It is worth recalling that thickening will occur in fascia in accordance with the degree of stress imposed upon it. Since enormous gravitational stress occurs in the abdominal region, as a result of postural embarrassment, it is frequently the case that tight 'stress bands' will be felt inferior, superior or lateral to internal organs (e.g. intestinal structures) that have sagged and become displaced. Such contracted tissue is often the source of reflex trigger activity and is often, in itself, the cause of mechanical interference with normal venous and lymphatic drainage, as well as being a possible source of pain. Any procedure that helps to normalise such tension should be accompanied by a programme of postural re-education and exercise if it is to have any lasting beneficial effects.

The operator's right hand, fingers flexed and middle finger slightly in the lead, probes through the surface abdominal musculature and attempts to 'lift' the structures. In this way, areas of abnormal resistance will be quite easily traced by the tip of the middle finger of the right hand. The most inferior point of attachment of such a band is located and held firmly by this flexed digit. The tip and lateral border of the thumb of the left hand is then placed adjacent to this contact, so that the right hand contact is on the tension band and the left contact is on the structure to which it attaches. The manipulative force is achieved by a rapid, anticlockwise movement of the right contact whilst firm, stabilising pressure is maintained by the left thumb.

The closer the two contacts are to each other at the moment of release, the less force is required and the less danger of injury to the tissues there will be. It is suggested that by visualising an attempt to tear an envelope held between thumbs and forefingers this concept will be better understood. The closer the holding digits are to each other the easier such an operation would be. Since the manipulative effort is attempting to, at least, stretch and, at most, separate the fibres involved, it is necessary to impart a high velocity, low amplitude torsional force and not a vague stretching effort imparted over a large area of unyielding tissue.

The actual manipulative force is imparted by the tip of the middle finger of the right hand but is of course the result of the movement of the whole hand. The wrist snaps medially and the elbow outwards at the moment of release. This speedy 'flicking' action is one that should be practised over and over again so that its execution is a matter of routine. A release of contracted tissue will be followed by an immediate freedom of mobility of tissues and of organs formerly 'bound' and immobile.

Such 'release' procedures (techniques A or B) should be performed throughout the abdominal area and should be preceded by the general neuromuscular treatment (p. 105) and be followed by a general procedure to 'lift' the abdominal contents back to a physiologically correct position. Abdominal and postural exercises on the part of the patient, combined with diaphragmatic breathing techniques, should also be carried out.

A series of six to ten such treatments over a period of a month or so is suggested in chronic conditions involving visceroptosis and abdominal congestion. The application of these techniques to the hypogastric and inguinal regions will be found to be of immense benefit to patients suffering from menstrual irregularities. Local function can be greatly improved as a result of the structural and circulatory improvements following specific release techniques.

Strain–counterstrain/positional release techniques (Fig. 8.14)
(Jones 1963, 1977)

In spinal and appendicular strains, injuries or lesions there is often an evident distortion from the normal anatomical posture or position. This eccentric state is often relieved by placing the

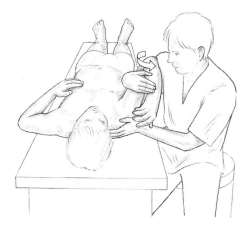

Figure 8.14B   A degree of ease is produced from that point by the initial positioning of the arm.

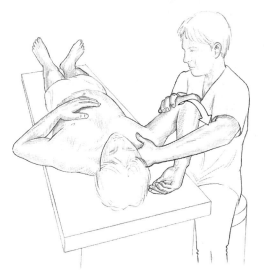

Figure 8.14C   A final position of ease is found by fine tuning to relieve pain in the tender point and the position is held for 20–90 seconds.

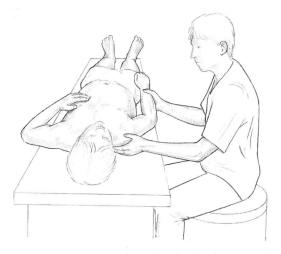

Figure 8.14A   A tender point is identified by the operator's left hand.

Figure 8.14   Application of positional release (strain/counterstrain) to the supraspinatus muscle.

joint or patient in an exaggerated degree of the deformity found at examination. If this is held for 90 to 120 seconds, a spontaneous release will often occur. Jones states that this technique depends on the ability to produce relaxation of reflex muscle tension which limits and binds the joint(s).

The art lies in finding the specific direction in which a painful joint can be moved which will release muscular tension as well as relieve pain. When passively placed in such a position, marked inhibition of painful stimuli will result and the range of motion of the area will usually be significantly enhanced subsequently. There are two mechanisms thought to be involved in the resolution of hypertonicity when strain/counterstrain is used: a neurological resetting involving the muscle spindles and a circulatory 'flushing' of previously ischaemic tissues (Rathbun et al 1970).

Jones' tender points

Jones has compiled lists of specific tender point areas relating to every imaginable strain of most joints and many muscles of the body. These are his 'proven' (by clinical experience) points and he provides strict guidelines for achieving ease in the tender point which is being palpated (position of ease usually involves a 'folding' or crowding of the tissues in which the tender point lies). A number of variations exist as to the use of the concepts which Jones developed and these are fully explained in a separate text in the series of which this book is part (*Positional Release Techniques*).

Tensor fascia lata (iliotibial band) techniques

The iliotibial band, when contracted or pathologically tight, is often misdiagnosed as a sacroiliac problem. The symptoms associated with its dysfunction may include pain, localised in the region of the medial or posterior superior iliac spine. There may be radiating pain to the anterior, lateral or posterior aspects of the thigh, and also in the iliac fossa, which may suggest

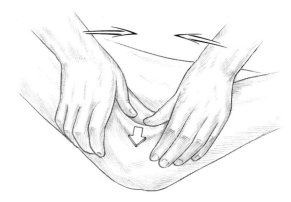

Figure 8.15A Anterior iliotibial band treatment, using a 'twig snapping' approach to address extreme shortness and fibrosity of these tissues. This is applied sequentially up and down the band using a degree of force which is easily tolerated.

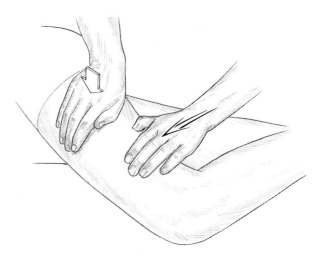

Figure 8.15B The posterior fibres of the iliotibial band are treated using the heel of one hand to alternately thrust against the band while it is stabilised by the other hand. An alternating sequence of this sort, applied up and down the band, produces marked release of hypertonic and shortened fibres.

visceral disease. The symptoms frequently arise in the sacroiliac joint, but its dysfunction is the result, in many cases, of tightness in the iliotibial band, the tissues of which may have numerous trigger points present.

One test for a tight iliotibial band is to have the patient lie on the unaffected side, with hip and knee flexed to 90°. The patient is asked to hold the knee down to the table. The other leg is taken by the operator, who is standing behind the patient. The leg is abducted and extended, to the point where the iliotibial band lies over the greater trochanter. The operator's cephalad hand will be palpating this structure, as the caudad hand raises and extends the suspected limb. The operator slides his caudad hand down so that the leg is supported only at the ankle, and the knee is flexed, thus allowing the knee to fall towards the table. If the iliotibial band has shortened this will not occur, but the leg will remain suspended. The band will palpate as tender under such conditions, as a rule.

Method 1. Treatment may employ a direct approach, as advocated by Mennell (1969) or by use of MET methods:

(a) Firstly the patient is placed side-lying, with both legs flexed comfortably. The first contact is with that part of the band distal to the greater trochanter. The anterior fibres are stretched first in a manner similar to that which would be used were the hands attempting to snap a stick (Fig. 8.15A). The fingers are laid over the anterior fibres of the band, distal to the trochanter, just above the knee. The thumbs rest, as a fulcrum, and are placed against the posterior aspect of the anterior fibres, and the snapping action is achieved by a rapid ulnar deviation of the hands (away from each other). The main force is transmitted through the thumbs, which should stretch the fibres without pressing them against the osseous structures (this would bruise the tissues). A series of movements such as this, starting at the knee and working upwards, is carried out.

(b) The posterior fibres are then treated. The heel of each hand is pushed in a piston-like manner against the fibres alternately. As the heel of one hand pushes against the fibres, the other stabilises them by grasping the anterior aspect (Fig. 8.15B). A series of thrusts are made from above the knee to the trochanter. Again the thrust must be against the fibres and not against osseous structures.

(c) The region overlying the trochanter is treated by rolling it backwards and forwards over the bony prominence. The thumbs are the motive force, being pressed downwards and

backwards, to achieve this. The roll is attempting to take the band posteriorly, over the trochanter. In order to roll it forward again, the middle fingers are employed. As it rolls backwards, the heel of the foot on the treated leg should rise from the table (but only if the band is tight).

(d) The area above the trochanter is treated by deep, kneading massage or NMT. This is often easily achieved when the patient is prone, and the tissues are contacted by the fingers of the treating hand, with the operator standing on the side opposite the area being treated. The fingers may be insinuated into the tissues, and a degree of lifting, drag, as well as pressure medialwards, is achieved by the operator leaning backwards and drawing the treating hand towards him. This may be done as part of NMT treatment. These structures require maintenance stretching, via exercise, if improvement is to be held.

Method 2. This involves either isometric or isolytic contraction.

Isometric contraction. In the first instance the patient is supine, with the unaffected leg flexed, and the affected leg extended. The operator takes the extended leg into maximum adduction, placing a maximum degree of stretch onto the lateral fibres (the abductors and fascia). In order to achieve this, the leg will be brought under the other, flexed, leg. Standing on the side of the unaffected leg and facing the patient, the operator takes out the slack, and asks the patient to make an attempt to abduct the affected leg. This is resisted for 10 seconds as the patient inhales. Release coincides with exhalation, at which time a little more slack is taken out and the affected leg is adducted slightly beyond its resistance barrier. The procedure is repeated two or three more times.

Isolytic contraction. The position is the same as above. Should the above be only partly effective, then, as the patient attempts to abduct the affected leg, (using only a portion – say 20% – of available strength) the operator overcomes this and forces it further into adduction. This might be uncomfortable, and the patient should be forewarned. This will produce microtrauma and reduce down fibrous contractions. Progressively more effort on the part of the patient should be introduced on subsequent isotonic eccentric contractions.

Trigger point techniques
(see also ischaemic compression and INIT above, pp. 113, 114 and Chapter 9)

There are a number of different pressure techniques used for dealing with trigger points. Where underlying (i.e. bony) tissues allow direct pressure onto such points, so that the trigger is squeezed between thumb and the underlying tissue, the variables will be the duration of such pressure and degree of continuous or variable pressure employed. Where no such suitable underlying tissues exist or where it would be dangerous to exert direct pressure through the muscle to the underlying structures (e.g. trigger points lying in sternocleidomastoid) then squeezing or pinching techniques can be employed. These will also vary as to the duration and nature (e.g. variable pressure) of the force imparted.

A combination of chilling and stretching of the tissues housing trigger points is known as 'spray and stretch' or chill-and-stretch technique treatment – this was discussed above (pp. 110–112).

Nimmo (1969) suggested a 5 to 7 second direct inhibitory pressure with a recheck of the tissues subsequently to assess reduced reflex activity.

The approach used until fairly recently by the principal author, was to apply a 5 second inhibitory pressure sufficient to reproduce the referred symptoms, followed by a short – 2 to 3 second – rest phase followed by a repeat of the initial pressure. This 'make and break' approach was continued until there was a reduction in the referred pain pattern intensity, or a significant alteration in the tone of the tissues, or until a minute or so had passed (with a cessation if the symptoms were intensifying rather than diminishing).

This was usually followed by an isometrically induced release of tone followed by stretching of the tissues housing the trigger point.

A more recent evolution involves use of an integrated neuromuscular inhibition technique (INIT) which is described in this chapter (p. 114) and in Chapter 9.

Chapman (Owen 1977) suggests a vibratory treatment, lasting 10 to 15 seconds, on the neurolymphatic reflexes that he described. He used fingertip pressure to impart the required energy, although thumb pressure of varying intensity is just as effective. This can be applied as a gradually intensifying pressure building up over 5 to 8 seconds, easing for 2 or 3 seconds and then repeated. Altogether this should not take more than half a minute. These points can be over-treated and the optimum time would seem to be from 15 to 30 seconds, with the pressure (or squeeze) of a variable nature.

It is important to realise that the objective 'feel' of local soft tissue contractions involving fibrosis is unlikely to change much during such treatment, whereas taut bands in which triggers lie frequently do 'release' (Baldry 1993). The main changes resulting from the treatment of fibrotic tissue will occur later, when homeostatic forces have come into operation. The variation in pressure during the treatment is more desirable than a constantly held degree of pressure, which may irritate and exacerbate the condition.

All the methods described in this chapter may be incorporated into general neuromuscular technique treatment.

REFERENCES

Abrams A 1922 New concepts in diagnosis and treatment. Physicoclinical Co., San Francisco

Acolet D 1993 Changes in plasma cortisol and catecholamine concentrations on response to massage in preterm infants. Archives of Disease in Childhood 68: 29–31

Baldry P 1993 Acupuncture, trigger points and musculoskeletal pain. Churchill Livingstone, Edinburgh

Castlio Y 1955 Effect of direct splenic stimulation in infectious diseases. American Academy of Osteopathy Yearbook 1955: 121

Chaitow B 1983 Personal communication to author.

Chaitow L 1990 Beat fatigue workbook. Thorsons, London

Chaitow L 1994 INIT in treatment of pain and trigger points. British Journal of Osteopathy XIII: 17–21

Chengnan S 1990 Chinese bodywork. Pacific View Press, Berkeley

Ferel-Torey A 1993 Use of therapeutic massage as a nursing intervention to modify anxiety and perceptions of cancer pain. Cancer Nursing 16(2): 93–101

Field T 1992 Massage reduces depression and anxiety in child and adolescent psychiatry patients. Journal of American Academy of Adolescent Psychiatry 31: 125–131

Fielding S 1983 Journal of Alternative Medicine December: 10–11

Hoag J 1969 Osteopathic medicine. McGraw Hill, New York, pp 189, 199

Hovind H et al 1974 Effects of massage on blood flow in skeletal muscle. Scandinavian Journal of Rehabilitation Medicine 6: 74–77

Ironson G et al 1993 Relaxation through massage associated with decreased distress and increased serotonin levels. Touch Research Institute, University of Miami School of Medicine. Unpublished MS

Janda V 1990 Muscle function testing. Butterworths, London

Janda V 1992 Muscle and back pain. Physical Medicine Research Foundation presentation, Vancouver BC October 1992

Johnson A 1939 Principles and practice of drugless therapeutics. W Straube, Los Angeles

Jones L 1963 Foot treatment without hand trauma. Journal of the American Osteopathic Association January

Jones L 1977 Strain and counterstrain. Academy of Applied Osteopathy

Lewit K 1985 Manipulative therapy in rehabilitation of the motor system. Butterworths, London

Lewit K 1992 Manipulative therapy in rehabilitation of the locomotor system. Butterworths, London

Marsh M 1969 Lecture notes. London

Mennell J 1969 Joint pain. Little, Brown

Mennell J 1974 Therapeutic use of cold. Journal of the American Osteopathic Association 74(12)

Nimmo R 1969 Lecture notes. British College of Naturopathy and Osteopathy

Owen C 1977 An endocrine interpretation of Chapman's reflexes. Academy of Applied Osteopathy

Polstein B 1991 In: DiGiovanna E (ed.) Osteopathic approach to diagnosis and treatment. J B Lippincott, Philadelphia

Puustjarvi K et al 1990 Effects of massage in patients with chronic tension headaches. Acupuncture and Electrotherapeutics Research 15: 159–162

Rathbun J et al 1970 Microvascular pattern of rotator cuff. Journal of Bone and Joint Surgery 52: 540–553

Retzlaff E et al 1974 Piriformis muscle syndrome. Journal of American Osteopathic Association 173: 799–807

Sandler S 1983 The physiology of soft tissue massage. British Osteopathic Journal 15: 1–6

Sleszynski S et al 1993 Comparison of thoracic manipulation and incentive spirometry in prevention of postoperative atelactasis. Journal of American Osteopathic Association August: 834–845

Stoddard A 1969 Manual of osteopathic practice. Hutchinson Medical, London

Travell J 1952 Ethyl chloride spray for painful muscle spasm. Archives of Physical Medicine and Rehabilitation 33: 291–298

Travell J, Simons D 1983 Myofascial pain and dysfunction, (vol 1) Williams and Wilkins, Baltimore

Travell J, Simons D 1992 Myofascial pain and dysfunction, (vol 2) Williams and Wilkins, Baltimore

Walther D 1988 Applied kinesiology. SDC Systems, Pueblo

Weinrich S, Weinrich M 1990 Effect of massage on pain in cancer patients. Applied Nursing Research 3: 140–145

Xujian S 1990 Effects of massage and temperature on permeability of initial lymphatics. Lymphology 23: 48–50

Zhao-Pu W 1991 Acupressure therapy. Churchill Livingstone, Edinburgh

9

Integrated neuromuscular inhibition technique (INIT)

TRIGGER POINTS

Travell and Simons have demonstrated the clear connection between myofascial trigger point activity and a wide range of pain problems and sympathetic nervous system aberrations (Travell & Simons 1986). Melzack and Wall confirm that there are few chronic pain problems which do not have myofascial trigger point activity as a component, with these acting, in many instances, as prime maintaining factors of the pain (Melzack & Wall 1988).

Trigger (and other non-referring pain) points commonly lie in muscles which have been stressed in a variety of ways including postural imbalances (Barlow 1959, Goldthwaite 1949), congenital factors (warping of fascia via cranial distortions (Upledger 1983), short leg problems, small hemipelvis etc.), occupational or leisure overuse patterns (Rolf 1977), emotional states reflecting into the soft tissues (Latey 1986), referred/reflex involvement of the viscera producing facilitated segments paraspinally (Beal 1983, Korr 1976), and trauma.

The repercussions of trigger point activity go beyond simple musculoskeletal pain – take, for example, their involvement in hyperventilation, chronic fatigue and apparent pelvic inflammatory disease. Trigger point activity is particularly prevalent in the muscles of the neck/shoulder region which also act as accessory breathing muscles. In situations of increased anxiety the incidence of borderline or frank hyperventilation is frequent (Bass et al 1985) and may be associated with chronic fatigue. Clinically these muscles palpate as tense, often fibrotic, with active trigger points being common (Roll et al 1987). Successful breathing retraining and normalisation of energy levels seem in such cases to be accelerated and enhanced following initial normalisation of the functional integrity of the involved muscles.

Slocumb (1984) has shown that in a large proportion of chronic pelvic pain problems in women, often destined for surgical intervention, the prime cause involves trigger point activity in muscles of the lower abdomen, perineum, inner thigh and even on the walls of the vagina.

Local facilitation

According to Korr (1976), a trigger point is a localised area of somatic dysfunction which behaves in a facilitated manner, i.e. it will amplify and be affected by any form of stress imposed on the individual whether this is physical, chemical or emotional. A trigger point is palpable as an indurated, localised, painful entity with a reference (target) area to which pain or other symptoms are referred (Chaitow 1991a).

Muscles housing trigger points can frequently be identified as being unable to achieve their normal resting length using standard muscle evaluation procedures (Janda 1983). The trigger point itself commonly lies in fibrotic tissue, which has evolved as the result of exposure of the tissues to diverse forms of stress.

Treatment methods

A wide variety of treatment methods have been advocated in treating trigger points, including inhibitory (ischaemic compression) pressure methods (Lief 1989, Nimmo 1966) acupuncture and/or ultrasound (Kleyhans and Aarons 1974), chilling and stretching of the muscle in which the trigger lies (Travell & Simons 1986), procaine or xylocaine injections (Slocumb 1984), active or passive stretching (Lewit 1992), and even surgical excision (Dittrich 1954).

Clinical experience, confirmed by the diligent research of Travell and Simons, has shown that

while all or any of these methods can successfully inhibit trigger point activity short-term, more is often needed to completely eliminate the noxious activity of the structure.

Common sense as well as clinical experience dictates that the next stage of correction of such problems should involve re-education (postural, breathing, relaxation etc.) or elimination of factors which contributed to the problem's evolution. This might well involve ergonomic evaluation of home and workplace as well as re-education methods mentioned above.

Travell and Simons have also shown that whatever initial treatment is offered to inhibit the neurological over-activity of the trigger point, the muscle in which it lies has to be made capable of reaching its normal resting length following such treatment or else the trigger point will rapidly reactivate.

In treating trigger points the method of chilling the offending muscle (housing the trigger) while holding it at stretch in order to achieve this end, was advocated by Travell and Simons, while Lewit has espoused the muscle energy method of a physiologically induced postisometric relaxation (or reciprocal inhibition) response, prior to passive stretching. Both methods are commonly successful, although a sufficient degree of failure occurs (trigger rapidly reactivates or fails to completely 'switch off') to require investigation of more successful approaches.

One reason for failure may relate to the possibility of the tissues which are being stretched not being the precise ones housing the trigger point.

A popular method for achieving tonus release in a muscle prior to stretching, involves introduction of an isometric contraction to the affected muscle (producing postisometric relaxation) or to its antagonist (producing reciprocal inhibition) (Chaitow 1991b).

The original use of isometric contractions prior to stretching was in proprioceptive neuromuscular facilitation techniques (PNF) which emerged from physical medicine in the early part of the 20th century. In most forms of muscle energy technique (MET) methodology, derived from osteopathic research and clinical experience, a partial (not full strength) isometric contraction is performed prior to the stretch in order to preclude tissue damage or stress to the patient and/or therapist which PNF quite frequently produces (Greenman 1989, Hartman 1985).

Hypothesis

The author hypothesises that partial contraction (using no more than 20 to 30% of patient strength, as is the norm in MET procedures) may sometimes fail to achieve activation of the fibres housing the trigger point being treated, since light contractions of this sort fail to recruit more than a small percentage of the muscle's potential.

Subsequent stretching of the muscle may only marginally involve the critical tissues surrounding and enveloping the myofascial trigger point.

Failure to actively stretch the muscle fibres in which the trigger is housed may account for the not infrequent recurrence of trigger point activity in the same site following treatment. Repetition of the same stress factors which produced it in the first place could undoubtedly also be a factor in such recurrence – which emphasises the need for re-education in rehabilitation.

A method which achieved precise targeting of these tissues (in terms of tonus release and subsequent stretching) would be advantageous.

Selye's concepts

Selye has described the progression of changes in tissue which is being locally stressed. There is an initial alarm (acute inflammatory) stage followed by a stage of adaptation or resistance when stress factors are continuous or repetitive, at which time muscular tissue becomes progressively fibrotic, and, if this change is taking place in muscle which has a postural rather than a phasic function, the entire muscle structure will shorten (Janda 1985, Selye 1984).

Clearly such fibrotic tissue, lying in altered (shortened) muscle, cannot simply 'release' itself in order to allow the muscle to achieve its normal resting length (as we have seen, this is a prerequisite of normalisation of trigger point activity). Along with various forms of stretch

(passive, active, MET, PNF etc.) it has been noted above that inhibitory pressure is commonly employed in treatment of trigger points.

Such pressure technique methods (analogous to acupressure or shiatsu methodology) are often successful in achieving at least short-term reduction in trigger point activity and are variously dubbed 'neuromuscular techniques' (Chaitow 1991c).

Application of inhibitory pressure may involve elbow, thumb, finger or mechanical pressure (a wooden rubber tipped T-bar is commonly employed in the US) or cross–fibre friction.

INIT HYPOTHESIS
(Chaitow 1994)

Clinical experience indicates that by combining the methods of direct inhibition (pressure mildly applied, continuously or in a 'make and break' pattern) along with the concept of strain/counterstrain and MET, a specific targeting of dysfunctional soft tissues can be achieved.

Strain/counterstrain (SCS) briefly explained

Jones (1981) has shown that particular painful 'points' relating to joint or muscular strain, chronic or acute, can be used as 'monitors' – pressure being applied to them as the body or body part is carefully positioned in such a way as to remove or reduce the pain felt in the palpated point.[1]

When the position of ease is attained (using what is known as 'fine tuning' in SCS jargon) in which pain vanishes from the palpated monitoring tender point, the stressed tissues are felt to be at their most relaxed – and clinical experience indicates that this is so since they palpate as 'easy' rather than having a sense of being 'bound' or tense.

---

[1]These tender points, as described by Jones, are found in tissues which were short rather than being stretched at the time of injury (acute or chronic) and are usually areas in which the patient was unaware of pain previous to their being palpated. They seem to equate in most particulars with 'ah shi' points in traditional Chinese medicine.

SCS is thought to achieve its benefits by means of an automatic resetting of muscle spindles – which help to dictate the length and tone in the tissues. This resetting apparently occurs only when the muscle housing the spindle is at ease and usually results in a reduction in excessive tone and release of spasm. When positioning the body (part) in strain/counterstrain methodology a sense of 'ease' is noted as the tissues reach the position in which pain vanishes from the palpated point.

INIT methods

Method 1 (see Fig. 9.1). It is reasonable to assume, and palpation confirms, that when a trigger point is being palpated by direct finger or thumb pressure, and when the very tissue in which the trigger point lies is positioned in such a way as to take away the pain (entirely or at least to a great extent), that the most (dis)stressed fibres in which the trigger point is housed are in a position of relative ease.

We would then have a trigger point under direct inhibitory pressure (mild or perhaps intermittent)

which had been positioned so that the tissues housing it are relaxed (relatively or completely).

Following a period of 20 to 30 seconds of this position of ease and inhibitory pressure – if the patient is asked to introduce an isometric con-

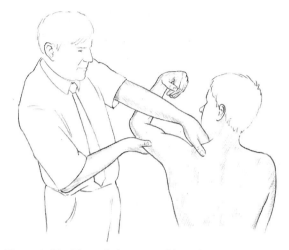

Figure 9.1B The pain is removed from the tender/pain/trigger point by finding a position of ease which is held for at least 20 seconds, following which an isometric contraction is achieved involving the tissues which house the tender/pain/trigger point.

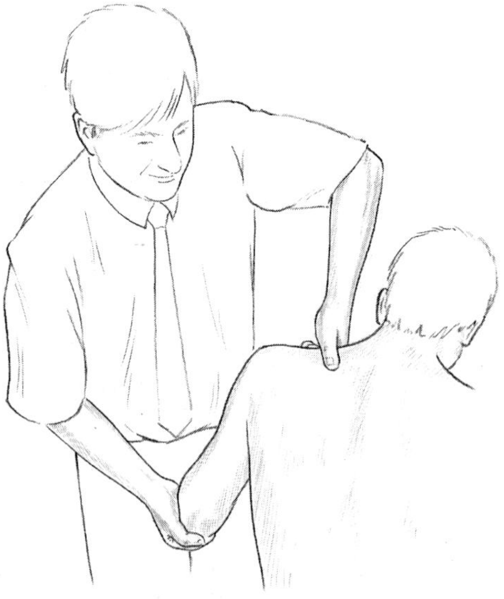

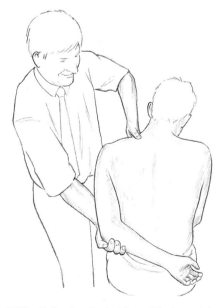

Figure 9.1A First stage of INIT in which a tender/pain/trigger point in supraspinatus is located and ischaemically compressed, either intermittently or persistently.

Figure 9.1C Following the holding of the isometric contraction for an appropriate period, the muscle housing the point of local soft tissue dysfunction is stretched. This completes the INIT sequence.

traction into the tissues and to hold this for 7 to 10 seconds – involving the very fibres which had been repositioned to obtain the strain/counterstrain release – there would subsequently occur a degree of reduction in tone in these tissues (postisometric relaxation). These could then be gently stretched as in any muscle energy procedure with the strong likelihood that specifically involved fibres would be stretched.

Method 2. There is another possibility – a variation in which, instead of an isometric contraction followed by stretch being commenced following the period of ease (strain/counterstrain position), an isolytic approach could be used.

The muscle receiving attention is actively contracted by the patient at the same time that a stretch is introduced – resulting in mild trauma to the muscle and the breakdown of fibrous adhesions between it and its interface and within its structures (Mitchell et al 1979).

To introduce this method into trigger point treatment, following the application of inhibitory pressure and SCS release, the patient is asked to contract the muscles around the palpating thumb or finger (lying on the now inhibited pain point) with the request that the contraction should not be a full strength effort since the operator intends to gently stretch the tissues while the contraction is taking place.

This isotonic eccentric effort – designed to reduce contractions and break down fibrotic tissue – should target precisely the tissues in which the trigger point being treated lies buried. Following the isolytic stretch the tissues could benefit from effleurage and/or hot and cold applications to ease local congestion. An instruction should be given to avoid active use of the area for a day or so.

Summary and comment

The integrated use of inhibitory pressure, strain/counterstrain and a form of muscle energy technique – applied to a trigger point or other area of soft tissue dysfunction involving pain or restriction of range of motion (of soft tissue origin), is a logical approach, since it has the advantage of allowing precise targeting of the culprit tissues.

Clearly the use of an isolytic approach as part of this sequence will be more easily achieved in some regions rather than others – upper trapezius posing less of a problem in terms of positioning and application than might quadratus lumborum.[2]

---

[2]No claim of absolute originality is made for this integrated approach which has evolved out of years of the author teaching the elements of it separately in the USA and Europe.

REFERENCES

Barlow W 1959 Anxiety and muscle tension pain. British Journal of Clinical Practice 13(5)
Bass C et al 1985 Respiratory abnormalities in chronic symptomatic hyperventilation. British Medical Journal 11 May 1985: 1387–1390
Beal M 1983 Palpatory testing of somatic dysfunction. Journal of American Osteopathic Association July
Chaitow L 1991a Palpatory literacy. Thorsons, London
Chaitow L 1991b Soft tissue manipulation. Thorsons, London
Chaitow L 1991c Soft tissue manipulation. Thorsons, London
Chaitow L 1994 INIT in treatment of pain and trigger points. British Journal of Osteopathy XIII: 17–21
Dittrich R 1954 Somatic pain and autonomic concomitants. American Journal of Surgery
Goldthwaite J 1949 Essentials of body mechanics. J B Lippincott, Philadelphia
Greenman P 1989 Manual medicine. Williams and Wilkins, Baltimore
Hartman L 1985 Handbook of osteopathic technique. Hutchinson, London
Janda V 1983 Muscle function testing. Butterworths, London
Janda V 1985 In: Glasgow E (ed.) Aspects of manipulative therapy. Churchill Livingstone, Edinburgh
Jones L 1981 Strain/counterstrain. Academy of Applied Osteopathy Colorado Springs
Kleyhans and Aarons 1974 Digest of Chiropractic Economics September
Korr I 1977 Spinal cord as organiser of the disease process. 1976 Yearbook Academy of Applied Osteopathy
Latey P 1986 Muscular manifesto. Published privately, London
Lewit K 1992 Manipulation in rehabilitation of the locomotor system. Butterworths, London

Lief S 1989 Described in: Chaitow L Neuro-muscular technique/soft tissue manipulation. Thorsons, Wellingborough

Melzack R, Wall P 1988 The challenge of pain. Penguin, London

Mitchell F, Moran P, Pruzzo N 1979 Evaluation of osteopathic muscle energy procedure. Valley Park

Nimmo R 1966 Receptor tonus technique. Lecture notes, London

Rolf I 1977 The Integration of human structures. Harper & Row, USA

Roll M et al 1987 Acute chest pain without obvious cause before age 40. Journal of Psychosomatic Research 31(2): 15–21

Selye H 1984 The stress of life. McGraw-Hill, USA

Slocumb J 1984 Neurological factors in chronic pelvic pain, trigger points and abdominal pelvic pain. American Journal of Obstetrics and Gynaecology 49: 536

Travell J, Simons D 1986 Trigger point manual. Williams and Wilkins, Baltimore

Upledger J 1983 Craniosacral therapy. Eastland Press, USA

10

NMT in clinical use

Wherever possible and useful, statements made in this text have carried citation references. Those statements not referenced represent the personal opinion of the author, based on 35 years of clinical experience as an osteopathic and naturopathic practitioner, in both private and National Health Service settings, in office practice and residential clinic settings, in Britain, Greece and the USA.

EVALUATION BEFORE TREATMENT

If therapeutic intervention is to be structured and organised and something other than hit-and-miss, there is an absolute requirement for sound evaluation and assessment as to the causes, extent and possible influences on other areas/tissues, of patterns of pain and restriction such as myofascial trigger points, locally traumatised areas, shortened and/or weakened muscles, joint restrictions and/or general/systemic factors (such as exist in arthritic conditions, for example).

NMT provides one such diagnostic/assessment tool and also offers, by switching from its assessment to its actively therapeutic mode, a means whereby very precisely focused and modulated degrees of force can be directed towards influencing restricted tissues, directly or reflexively. Myofascial release techniques, as well as ischaemic compression (osteopathic inhibitory technique), can be applied to precise targets via the contacting thumb or finger in NMT.

Perhaps NMT's greatest usefulness in assessment relates to the opportunity it offers for the identification of local soft tissue dysfunction in a gentle, non-invasive manner. In the USA as well as in the UK, the focus of many therapists utilising NMT is primarily on myofascial trigger points (and the often widespread musculo-skeletal dysfunction which produces them) and in order to utilise NMT to its full advantage, it is necessary to have a clear understanding of the process of facilitation which can occur para-spinally or locally in muscle and fascia (trigger points) as described in detail in Chapter 3 (p. 30).

By learning how to use NMT diagnostically and therapeutically, a good deal of information can be obtained as to the patterns of dysfunction operating. It is important to stress once more that NMT may be used in both a diagnostic mode and a therapeutic mode, and that to some extent these overlap, and may be carried out simultaneously. Once having identified those structures and tissues which required greater attention, NMT is available as a tool with which to make contact and give direct localised treatment to areas which are contracted or tightened. Specific techniques are also available to deal with reflex activity, such as is noted in trigger points. Muscle energy methods, as described by Lewit, and elaborations on these, derived from a variety of sources, provide a further array of techniques which can be brought into operation, depending upon the particular indications. Many of these associated techniques were described in Chapter 8.

What about joints?
(Chaitow 1983, 1991, Jones 1981, Mitchell et al 1979)

Soft tissue manipulation, which includes positional release methods ('strain/counterstrain') NMT and MET, is capable of normalising a great many joint problems, without recourse to active manipulative effort. MET and NMT are symbiotic, and it is possible to achieve more by combining their repertoire of useful techniques, than either can achieve individually. By adding the knowledge of suitable techniques by which to influence reflex activity, demonstrated by the presence of localised areas of soft tissue dysfunction (trigger points, Chapman's points, localised fibrosis etc.) as well as by using the tender points described by Jones, in gentle functional techniques, the scope of soft tissue manipulation methods should become apparent.

Employment of these approaches does not necessarily preclude the need for active joint manipulation in correcting restriction but can make for a lesser need to utilise high velocity thrusts or long lever techniques, and to make their employment simpler, and far less likely to traumatise the local tissues or the patient.

Avoiding trauma

By combining MET and NMT, some degree of the potential problem of tissue damage is likely to be solved. NMT, applied to a region containing fibrotic change, will allow for subsequent use of 'normal' MET, or of an isolytic contraction, with less discomfort or likelihood of microtrauma (see Chapter 8, p. 114).

Are some musculoskeletal problems best left untreated?

The enormous privilege which the patient allows, in permitting the practitioner to make physical contact, also grants a degree of 'power' to the operator. Defences are lowered, and the patient is likely to be amenable to discussing areas of their emotions and thoughts, which they might resist in other situations. This presents opportunities for therapeutic intervention on other levels than the physical. The operator should be aware of the potent 'placebo' effect which such a situation allows. Suggestions, and positive guidance, can have powerful influences on the patient, and so care should be exercised, and diligent application of healing techniques undertaken, knowing that the recipient is, as a rule, receptive and highly suggestible.

When considering treatment of soft tissue changes which, to a large extent, involve emotional inputs, it is important to realise the need for an adequate ability on the part of the practitioner/therapist to handle any emotional repercussions resulting from 'releasing' (or attempting to release) the soft tissue manifestations of emotional turmoil, or to have an adequate referral system in place to support the patient in times of need.

If the patient himself is not capable of processing whatever emotional baggage is attached to a particular pattern of soft tissue dysfunction, then it is probably best left intact, until the patient is ready and equipped to handle the issues which are submerged in his physical state.

A scenario is conceivable in which a patient with obvious musculoskeletal dysfunction but without obvious mento-emotional problems, could be left in a fragile and vulnerable state following apparently appropriate bodywork. The oft-quoted phenomenon of 'emotional release' which occurs during or following treatment may be something which therapists could usefully reflect upon and possibly re-evaluate. Just how beneficial, or how dangerous, is such a reaction without further support such as counselling or psychotherapy?

Lief's methods

Stanley Lief, the prime developer of NMT, employed few specific manipulative techniques. His main concern was to attempt to normalise mobility and function (circulation, drainage, nerve function, etc.) and, to this end, his neuromuscular treatment was often accompanied by no more than general rotary movements of the cervical and lumbar areas together with a degree of 'springing' or stretching of the dorsal region. Derision on the part of the 'specific' manipulators should be tempered by the fact that this general, 'constitutional' treatment approach (some would call it 'engine wiping') achieves phenomenal results in terms of improvement in general wellbeing and the alleviation of many specific lesion patterns.

Undoubtedly there exist specific spinal and joint problems that require an individual approach; however, the correction of the supporting mechanisms (muscles, fascia, ligaments, tendons) via NMT on its own or together with general mobilising techniques of soft tissue manipulation, is able to frequently obviate the need for any more detailed technique. Indeed, specific 'adjusting' of joints, which pays no heed to the soft tissue component, is far more likely to fail (in the sense that symptoms speedily return) than the Lief method.

Speransky and Selye: common findings
(Selye 1976, Speransky 1943)

The final conclusion, which Speransky offers us, and which is pertinent to acupuncture and all methods of physical treatment, is the following: 'Hence we obtain the rule that only weak degrees of irritation can have a useful significance; strong ones inevitably do damage.'

These words should be locked in the minds of all therapists, of whatever school. The term 'irritation', is used by Speransky, and this is of interest, since a little thought will indicate that whatever is being done to a patient, in terms of therapy, involves to a greater or lesser extent an element of stress (or irritation) – stress, in this sense, being defined as any stimulus, pleasant or unpleasant, which calls upon the body to respond, or adapt, in some manner.

Manipulation, acupuncture, pressure techniques, use of heat and cold, hydrotherapy, electrical and mechanical therapies, surgery, and indeed the whole gamut of medications, whether they be drugs or homoeopathic dilutions of herbal substances – all call for a response on the part of the body. All are, therefore, to a degree, 'stress' factors. Speransky insists that only mild irritants can have a useful role to play in evoking a positive (i.e. healing) response.

Selye shows stress can be helpful

Hans Selye (1976) has come to precisely the same conclusion in his important research into stress. In experiments carried out in his extensive studies, Selye produced subcutaneous sacs in experimental animals by injecting a given volume of air under the skin. This was followed by the insertion of an irritant of some sort. He first demonstrated that the amount of exudate, and the thickness of the sac wall varied, as one might anticipate, with the strength and concentration of the irritant substance. He followed this by introducing a form of stress, such as intense cold, heat or forced immobilisation.

The response of the animals varied greatly. In those that had been initially injected with a weak irritant, the stress which was then added seemed to aid the recovery, as evidenced by resolution of the irritated area, and inhibition of tissue fibrosis. Those animals, however, which had had strong irritants injected into the subcutaneous sacs, responded to the subsequent stress factor by showing an increase in inflammation, widespread necrosis, and often death. Selye concluded with these words: 'This was the crucial experiment, showing that stress can either cure or aggravate a disease, depending upon whether the inflammatory response to a local irritant is necessary or superfluous.'

We now have Speransky's and Selye's combined evidence, that what we do to a patient, in terms of therapy, can be beneficial or harmful, and that this to a great extent will depend upon the degree of the irritation involved in the treatment, whatever form it takes.

Speransky's work further teaches us that Mann's words are true (see Chapter 3, p. 26), that *any part of the surface of the body* can be an initiator of a process involving neurological changes, which can be pathological or therapeutic. The classifying of certain points as being trigger points, others as being acupuncture alarm points, and yet others as being neurolymphatic or neurovascular – or any other – points, is merely a matter of convenience. It helps us to make a degree of sense out of the enormous amount of information available to us. That, to an extent, these points may be interchangeable, is obvious. For many are patently found in the self-same position, on different 'maps' of points. There are subtle variations in the behaviour of some points, such as has already been described with trigger points having a reference area (target area) and other points being found in pairs etc. This is a matter of practical classification, and interpretation of the characteristics

of different points. They are all to some extent interchangeable, however, and a latent trigger point, which may be identified as sensitive but with no referral capabilities, might become an active trigger by the simple introduction of a chill, or a strain, to that area. Bearing in mind therefore that the distinction between the points discussed is man-made, we will continue to classify them in these ways as a matter of convenience. It should also be borne in mind that whenever acupuncture points are mentioned, the availability of these for manual treatment (pressure, chilling, heating, etc.) remains. There is some evidence that needling can achieve particular effects, not available to pressure techniques, but this is equivocal, and for the purposes of soft tissue manipulation, pressure can usually be shown to be as effective as needling, with the one major drawback, that only a limited number of points can be contacted by hand at any one time, as compared with the multiple needling which is possible in acupuncture.

CORRECT SEQUENCE OF THERAPY

Treatment of dysfunction associated with muscles which have become weak could involve initial attention to their antagonists which may be inhibiting them, as well as use of isotonic concentric MET methods applied to weak muscles themselves, along with exercises specific to the area. General postural and body-toning exercises should follow. Before such exercise is initiated it is important to discover and treat local dysfunction within shortened or weakened muscles – such as trigger points – and NMT will usefully achieve this. It may then be useful to allow the beneficial effects of the attention to the shortened muscles to proceed without confusing the issue by exercising the weakened antagonists. If, after several weeks of treatment of the shortened, contracted, postural muscles and their trigger points, there is not an observable and measurable improvement in the weak antagonists, then MET and exercise should be introduced to these. The use of gentle functional techniques, such as those of Jones (strain/counterstrain, for example) are suitable for combining with NMT and MET methods. By using muscle energy techniques, to help to lengthen shortened structures, and NMT to aid in this, as well as in identifying localised areas of soft tissue dysfunction (myofascial trigger points or other forms of soft tissue dysfunction) the therapist/practitioner has a wide array of diagnostic and therapeutic methods, literally at his finger tips.

Massage

We should not lose sight of the tried and tested effects of massage on the soft tissues. The degree of that effect will vary with the type of soft tissue manipulation employed, and the nature of the patient and the problem.

Soft tissue techniques, apart from those specifically associated with NMT, may include:

- Stroking (to include relaxation and reduce fluid congestion).
- Stretching (along or across the belly of muscles. Heel of hand, thumb or fingers are involved in slow movements, rhythmically applied).
- Inhibition via pressure (directly applied to the belly or origins or insertions of contracted muscles or to local soft tissue dysfunction, for a minute or more, or in a make and break manner, to reduce hypertonic contraction or for reflex effect).
- Kneading (to improve fluid exchange and to achieve relaxation of tissues).
- Vibration and friction (used near origins and insertions, and near bony attachments, for relaxing effects on the muscle as a whole).

Other methods which we would associate with the above techniques of traditional massage (soft tissue manipulation) would include the various applications of NMT, as described in this text, and connective tissue massage methods which are primarily used for reflex effects. See Chapters 4, 5 and 8 for details of these methods.

Effects explained

How are the various effects of massage and soft tissue manipulation explained? Sandler (1983) believes that a combination of effects occur.

Pressure, as applied in deep kneading or stroking along the length of a muscle, tends to displace its fluid content. Venous, lymphatic and tissue drainage is thereby encouraged. The replacement of this with fresh oxygenated blood, aids in achieving homeostatic balance, and reduces the effects of pain-inducing substances which may be present via increased capillary filtration and reduction in oedema. Venous capillary pressure is also increased by massage. Massage is thought to produce a decrease in the sensitivity of the gamma efferent control of the muscle spindles, thereby reducing any shortening tendency of the muscles. Pressure techniques, such as are used in NMT, and the methods employed in MET, have a direct effect on the Golgi tendon organs, which detect the load applied to the tendon or muscle. These have an inhibitory capability, which can cause the entire muscle to relax. The Golgi tendon organs are set in series in the muscle, and are affected by both active and passive contraction of the tissues. The effect of any system which applies longitudinal pressure or stretch to the muscle, will be to evoke this reflex relaxation. The degree of stretch has, however, to be great, as there is little response from a small degree of stretch. The effect of MET, articulation techniques, and various functional balance techniques depends to a large extent on these tendon reflexes (Sandler 1983).

Lewit's view

We are in the midst of a change in the concepts of manipulative therapy which has far-reaching implications. One of the major changes is the restoration of the soft tissue component to centre stage, rather than the peripheral role to which it has been assigned in the past. Lewit (1985) discusses aspects of this. He describes the 'no man's land', which lies between neurology, orthopaedics and rheumatology which, he says, is the home of the vast majority of patients with pain derived from the locomotor system, and in whom no definite pathomorphological changes are found. He makes the suggestion that these be termed cases of 'functional pathology of the locomotor system'. These include most of the patients attending osteopathic, chiropractic and physiotherapy practitioners.

The most frequent symptom of individuals involved in this area of dysfunction is pain, which may be reflected clinically by reflex changes such as muscle spasm, myofascial trigger points, hyperalgesic skin zones, periosteal pain points, or a wide variety of other sensitive areas which have no obvious pathological origin.

It is a major part of the role of NMT to help in both identifying such areas and offering some help in differential diagnosis. NMT and other soft tissue methods are then capable of normalising many of the causative aspects of these myriad and mysterious sources of pain and disability.

Ideals

The holistic, total, approach to the problems of human health is one which looks to the causes of dysfunction and disease and, by removing these, allows the homeostatic efforts of the body to restore normality. This ideal is not always attainable but it should remain the aim of the therapist. Each individual has an optimum degree of biomechanical (structural, postural, functional), biochemical and psychological efficiency that can be realised. It is this optimum that is being aimed for in all therapies that fall into the broad net of holistic healing methods.

NMT takes its place amongst these methods, since its objective is to help to restore the structural, functional and postural integrity of the body by removing restrictions and aiding in the normalisation of dysfunction. NMT aids the economy and functional ability of the body further by reducing self-perpetuating stress factors such as contractions, spasms and tensions in the soft tissue components of the system. By improving function, removing pain, reducing energy loss, improving posture etc., the effect on psychologically negative states is a positive one.

In itself NMT is only a tool, a useful method or technique which can be of immense use in a variety of conditions. It possesses one further criterion which places it firmly in the holistic 'tool box'. This is, that it does nothing to the body which is harmful to its overall state of health i.e. it has no side-effects. Indeed, by normalising the soft tissues, NMT often saves the individual from techniques of a more 'violent' nature which might well produce outward reactions, such as surgery, traction, immobilisation etc., and techniques which, whilst not usually harmful, can be painful, such as manipulative joint techniques.

NMT has an immense capability for diagnostic application, and since this can take place at the same time as its therapeutic application, it shows economy in the use of time and energy. Since NMT is entirely a manual technique it is not wasteful of resources such as heat, power etc. and is applicable under almost any circumstances or conditions.

When is NMT useful?

NMT may be universally applied to any patient of any age suffering from any condition. This is not to say that it will be curative, or even of marked value, in all conditions. But it will be of some diagnostic and some therapeutic value in every condition and of enormous value in others, since no one is free of some degree of dysfunction, affecting the overall efficiency and economy of the body.

In general terms, NMT may be applied to all cases of musculoskeletal dysfunction and mento-emotional dysfunction with benefit. The basic spinal and basic abdominal techniques are used as diagnostic and therapeutic tools in the majority of cases. The more specific techniques such as psoas, piriformis, TFL and abdominal release techniques are used as and when indicated. A general, full body NMT treatment may be applied as part of a programme of postural reintegration.

In specific terms, NMT is applied as follows. All conditions of the spine and conditions which involve the arms or legs would receive general spinal technique as well as consideration of local areas, in the limbs affected. Such treatments would be repeated once or twice weekly until a degree of normality had been achieved. As should be obvious, other modalities and techniques would and should be used if called for. NMT combines with anything of a supportive nature which is aimed at the restoration of normal function, such as (in appropriate conditions) ultrasonic therapy, diathermy, manipulation etc. At the outset, the aim of general treatment is to remove the more obvious areas of contraction and stasis. All reflex trigger points should be neutralised by pressure techniques if possible or, if found stubborn, by chill and stretch, MET or infiltration methods. As therapy progresses, individual patterns of dysfunction will become clear and more specific NMT would be applied to those spinal, abdominal, intercostal and pelvic areas slow to improve.

Manipulative techniques of a non-specific type are often useful in the normalisation of spinal integrity once the initial soft tissue rigidity or dysfunction has been improved. NMT may be applied with infinite gentleness or with robust enthusiasm, since it is possible to use the same techniques with a marked difference in the degree of force employed. This enables its application to areas of acute sensitivity as well as in fragile (osteoporotic) and tender areas. As long as the operator is thinking about the task in hand and not applying the techniques in a mechanical, repetitive manner, there is no danger of injury or harm.

If treatment is aimed at the removal of symptoms stemming from trigger points, it is essential to normalise all the structures related to the local area of dysfunction. To simply neutralise the trigger that is causing, say, a headache, will produce short-term benefits. If the particular trigger lies in the trapezius muscle then not only must the trigger be normalised and the trapezius treated, but the entire cervical and spinal musculature and soft tissues must receive attention. A general rule should be that no part of the whole should be considered without the whole also being considered. Thus, even if the spinal areas are receiving the main attention of the therapist on any one visit, the muscles of the lower limb and associated structures should be given some consideration to assess their involvement and possible requirements. The treatment of the back, therefore, calls

for the treatment of the front and this calls for the whole to be considered and treated.

General abdominal technique is useful in all cases of digestive and intestinal dysfunction of a non-pathological nature. NMT is applicable to all cases of respiratory dysfunction. It is also applicable to all genitourinary conditions of a non-pathological nature. NMT applied to the abdomen will reduce dramatically many tension states of mento-emotional origin. General abdominal technique improves circulatory efficiency through the pelvis and abdominal regions and it improves respiratory function. The reflex points and zones in the spinal area should always be treated prior to thoracic and abdominal technique as indicated. In a case of spastic constipation, for example, NMT to the lower spinal areas and the use of neurolymphatic points followed by general abdominal technique would be the pattern recommended. This could be followed by specific abdominal release techniques if areas of marked contractions or 'adhesion' were elicited during the general treatment. In the author's experience, such an approach, combined with general health measures such as nutritional reform together with appropriate exercise and relaxation programmes, will promote a return to normal more speedily than anything else. If the body is being given those factors required for normality, its self-healing tendency, which is constantly acting, will respond positively to the removal of obstacles to recovery (structural, mechanical, dietary).

In dealing with tension and stress of psychic origin it is as well to recall that the mind will not be calm or relaxed as long as neuromuscular tensions are present. In applying any form of psychotherapy, the use of NMT, applied to the spine and abdomen, will increasingly improve the patient's ability to relax. NMT is not seen as an end in itself in this regard, but to be a catalyst to the removal or easing of the physical component of a vicious circle. In some cases this physical release of tension, especially when applied to the solar plexus, can produce a sudden emotional release in which the patient may cry and sob. The body becomes a solid mass of tensions and contractions for many individuals.

The tensions of life are mirrored by layers of muscular 'armour'. The posture and tensions thus created all carry specific emotional charges and memories and as the physical components are eased so do the emotional memories and feelings associated with their origins come to the surface. Just how appropriate it is to initiate such 'releases' was discussed earlier in this chapter (p. 144).

In restoring total structural and postural integrity to the body, it is necessary to apply NMT to all the supporting structures. This might involve the spinal, thoracic and abdominal soft tissues and the limbs, including the feet. NMT and manipulation, where appropriate, will lay the foundations for a return to normal (or to the patient's individual optimum norm). Specific and general exercise, as well as postural re-education, may then follow. It is possible, via such systems as Alexander technique, to achieve postural and functional normality. It is contended, however, that with the judicious use of NMT and soft tissue and, if necessary, osseous manipulation, such re-education becomes much easier and less arduous. It must be easier to learn to use a machine correctly if that machine is capable of functioning correctly!

The same proviso applies to breathing retraining. Unless the thoracic and diaphragmatic structures are to some extent made pliable by therapeutic interventions such as those detailed in earlier chapters, such retraining will of necessity involve struggling against great odds.

In attempting to achieve postural and functional normality, a fairly long-term view is required. Some workers assert that a series of eight to ten treatment sessions will produce this result. It is the author's experience that, whilst the basic ground work can be done in eight to ten treatments, the majority of cases require weekly or fortnightly treatment for 12 to 18 months if they are to achieve optimum improvement. This should be followed by maintenance visits at not less than 3 monthly intervals.

Just as retraining (posture, breathing) without appropriate bodywork is doomed to partial success at best, so bodywork methods which ignore retraining and re-education will have only short-term benefits, since much of any chronic dysfunctional pattern of use will be firmly locked into habitual neural and behavioural patterns.

Structural and functional changes are interdependent – they follow each other causally as well as therapeutically. NMT is universally applicable. It has no side-effects. It combines with all other methods of positive health care. In itself it is capable of improving general function, releasing tension and removing noxious triggers, which may be responsible for myriad symptoms. NMT has limits, but within the framework of its own area of application its only limits lie in the ability of the operator.

Moule's methods

One practitioner who has achieved outstanding success in applying NMT to athletic injuries of marked severity is Terry Moule. In the 1970s he restored the former captain of England's soccer team, Gerry Francis, to playing fitness. Surgery to the lumbar spine was the only prospect left for Francis after months of agony under orthopaedic investigation. In desperation Moule was consulted and within a few weeks Francis was playing again. He remains fit and continues to be involved in professional soccer as Tottenham Hotspur's manager.

A similar return to normality was achieved in the case of the then captain of England's rugby football team, Roger Uttley, whose career appeared to be over after a back injury. Treatment consisting largely of NMT resulted in Uttley returning to the England squad in their successful 1980 season.

An even more startling result of the application of NMT to a spinal injury involved then world mile and 1500 m record holder Sebastian Coe. He stated in late 1979: 'Last winter I had a back problem. I was having trouble getting a diagnosis, let alone treatment.' Within a few treatments incorporating NMT he was running again and setting world record times.

Terry Moule's view of NMT is as follows:

The principle of NMT is that it is of prime importance to treat connective tissue lesions and abnormalities, prior to any manipulative treatment of the bony structures. If more orthodox and less penetrating soft tissue techniques are used, whilst the bony abnormality may be corrected by the application of a specific adjustment, because the soft tissues remain in a similar state to that existing prior to the manipulation, there is a strong likelihood of a recurrence of the lesion. NMT tends to dispense with specific adjustment, for, subsequent to using these specialised soft tissue measures, a generalised mobilisation adjustment will allow the muscular and connective tissues to encourage the bony structures to return to their normal alignment. This may take a little longer to produce relief from discomfort, but in the long run it means that the correction is more permanent and there is less danger of any damage to the muscular and connective tissues from forceful manipulation.

The great advantage of NMT is that it may be applied to any part of the body. It is particularly effective in dealing with problems related to interference with nerve supply; to any form of muscular or connective tissue lesion; to treatment of the abdominal and pelvic organs etc. It is applied mainly by use of the thumb. It may take some years to develop an adequate 'feel' in the hands in general and the thumbs in particular, to effectively diagnose and treat lesions. It is the ability to diagnose through the thumb which is so helpful in the rapid and efficient treatment of all forms of dysfunction. Correctly used it precludes a large number of more conventional techniques and saves a considerable amount of time.

NMT has proved invaluable in the treatment of sports injuries, particularly for the diagnostic reasons outlined above and for the fact that it produces a rapid response as compared to orthodox soft tissue and physiotherapy techniques. With sports injuries one of the major problems is to get the player back in action as soon as possible, particularly where the injury is to a professional sportsman. NMT has been used very effectively on a large number of sportsmen and women following all types of sports.

One of the most common injuries one encounters is hamstring problems. These are particularly prevalent amongst footballers, who in many cases develop the injury through overdevelopment of the quadriceps without adequate attention to the maintenance and mobility (i.e. lengthening and stretching) of the hamstrings at the same time. The normal treatment of hamstring injuries is ultra-sonic and massage. These techniques are not particularly rapid and the resultant loss of overall muscle tone, due to the inability of the leg to be used normally, retards a return to normal function. With NMT a lesion can be accurately and rapidly detected and, by the use of deep thumb manipulation, the soft tissue lesion can be dealt with rapidly and effectively. Where there is muscular fibre

damage this can be felt and literally ironed out. The effect of the technique is to stimulate circulation in the area thus encouraging healing. Where there is inflammation and swelling the technique promotes drainage and the restoration of normal tone. With acute lesions the technique is unfortunately painful, but where speed is the prime order in recovery this is a small price to pay.

NMT is also beneficial in the treatment of knee lesions, particularly ligamentous problems and the subsequent inflammation in the joint itself. Correct application of NMT to these lesions will improve drainage from the knee and encourages healing to take place far more rapidly than through orthodox techniques. Where there is knee misalignments or dislocation, reduction of spasm is most important as a prerequisite to satisfactory manipulation of the joint. In many cases injury occurs when the legs become anchored due to studs in the boots. If rotation of the trunk is superimposed onto this static lower limb situation the stress imposed on the knee joint is enormous. The application of NMT prior to attempting correction not only makes the correction less painful but ensures that the result is lasting. NMT is also beneficial in the treatment of prepatellar bursitis, and any synovial inflammatory problems.

A problem which plagues many sportsmen, particularly footballers, basketball players and volleyball players, is pain in the groin and down the inside of the leg. This is commonly treated as a sacroiliac or a lumbar problem when, in many cases, it is due to a lesion of the symphysis-pubis. There are a number of techniques for dealing with problems of this joint but none so dramatically successful as the application of NMT.

The technique's effectiveness in producing long-term benefits is perhaps best underlined by the results with sportsmen such as Roger Uttley and Gerry Francis, who had both received short-term benefit from manipulative treatment. The application of NMT, without any change in the manipulative techniques being employed, except to make them less specific, produced long-term improvement which allowed a return to active participation in their respective sports. In both cases the main problem was an imbalance in muscle tone with excessive tension causing persistence of the joint dysfunction. The removal of these soft tissue factors restored balance and encouraged the body to return to normal function, as it always tries to do.

In summary, the benefits of NMT in general are (1) that it is a technique which removes causes rather than dealing with symptoms. (2) It removes the necessity for the bulk of specific manipulation, instead it encourages the body to normalise itself. (3) It is applicable to any part of the body. From the specific sports injury point of view the main advantage of NMT is that it provides (1) a more rapid recovery rate and (2) a more permanent one.

The author's own experience confirms the validity of Terry Moule's comments. NMT, apart from all the myriad applications discussed in earlier chapters, is the finest soft tissue system for helping to normalise acute and chronic injuries. In the past 35 years I have used these methods on tens of thousands of patients. In many cases sporting and theatrical performers have been restored to normal in a short space of time. Where the 'show must go on' – and in present terms this applies to athletic and sporting performance just as much as to theatrical performance – time is vital. NMT and the various methods that may accompany it, such as ultra-sonics, manipulation, hydrotherapy, exercise, cryotherapy etc., have been successful time after time. I have found NMT invaluable in dealing with acute injuries affecting major public and political figures in both the UK and Greece as well as such personalities as Richard Burton (acute torticollis during the filming of *Look Back in Anger*), James Booth (acute low back during the West End run of *Fings Aint What They Used To Be*), Christopher Neame (neck injury sustained in fall from balcony during *Romeo and Juliet*), Bryan Forbes (neck strained during filming of *League of Gentlemen*), Harry Andrews (who fell off a horse during filming *Devil's Disciple*).

All of these were able to resume work within 1 day of their injury. In all cases no proper treatment facilities were available. Conditions ranged from the dressing room floor for James Booth to the lush grass of Tring Park for Harry Andrews. No equipment was available other than my hands and no treatment was used other than NMT and gentle mobilisation. The economy, versatility and effectiveness of NMT has proved itself over and over again. In more chronic conditions, NMT has proved equally useful on countless occasions.

The successful use of NMT calls for the applied thought of the practitioner. The body responds rapidly to the help this technique offers. Its limitations are almost always related to the limitations of the practitioner. Its success is in direct proportion to the dedication and intelligence with which it is applied.

REFERENCES

Chaitow L 1983 Neuromuscular technique. Thorsons, London
Chaitow L 1991 Soft tissue manipulation. Healing Arts Press, Rochester, Vermont
Jones L 1981 Strain and counterstrain. Academy of Applied Osteopathy, Colorado Springs
Lewit K 1985 Manipulative therapy in rehabilitation of the motor system. Butterworths, London

Mitchell F, Moran P, Pruzzo N 1979 Evaluation of osteopathic muscle energy procedure. Valley Park
Sandler S 1983 The physiology of soft tissue massage. British Osteopathic Journal 15: 1–6
Selye H 1976 The stress of life. McGraw Hill, New York
Speransky 1943 A basis for the theory of medicine. International Publishers, New York

11

American neuromuscular therapy

Judith (Walker) DeLany LMT

History

As detailed in Chapter 2, neuromuscular therapy (NMT) evolved out of the work of a number of clinicians working in both Europe and the USA.[1] The American development of NMT (neuromuscular 'therapy' rather than neuromuscular 'technique', the preferred term in Europe) was largely based on the methods devised and taught by the late Raymond Nimmo, subsequently modified and expanded by Paul St John and Judith (Walker) DeLany.

Nimmo's research into the pathological influences and relevance, as well as the therapeutic implications of treating, 'noxious pain points', mirrors closely that of his contemporary, Janet Travell, in relation to her research into myofascial trigger points.

St John's work was initially based on that of Nimmo, with whom he had studied, as well as the writings and research of Travell & Simons (1983), Vannerson & Nimmo (1971), Calliet (1977) and others through their writings and seminars. St John's collaboration and teaching programmes, conducted with Judith (Walker) DeLany, resulted in revisions of previous concepts and methodology, leading to significant changes in recommended treatment techniques (see below).

---

[1] Variations existing between the European and American versions of NMT will be highlighted in this chapter by brief comments which are given in footnotes. The European version is commonly known as 'Lief's NMT', which is the way it will be described in these notes.

St John's teaching currently incorporates structural homeostasis of the body and cranium, while (Walker) DeLany takes a broader view which incorporates a systematic approach towards pain relief, involving attention to ischaemia, trigger points, nerve compression/entrapment, postural distortion (biomechanics), nutrition and emotional wellbeing (stress reduction). This introduction to NMT will concentrate on the basic technique and examples of application to selected muscles. There is no substitute for hands-on instruction and this is highly recommended as the only safe means of acquiring NMT skills.

Applications of NMT

In most applications of NMT, dry work, such as myofascial release or skin rolling, is performed first. This is followed by manipulation or lightly lubricated gliding aimed at increasing blood flow, 'flushing' tissues while at the same time evaluating for ischaemic bands and/or trigger points. Static digital or manual pressure is subsequently employed in order to release ischaemic bands and for treatment of trigger points, usually after several repetitions of gliding have been completed. Pressure bars may be used instead of, or in addition to, finger or thumb compression (see Fig. 11.1A,B).

Manually applied gliding is repeated after the application of compression or friction.

NMT TECHNIQUES

Gliding (effleurage) is an important and powerful component of neuromuscular therapy. It warms the fascia, flushes blood through the tissues and therefore increases oxygenation and perfusion of nutrients while simultaneously eliminating waste products from the tissues (Yates 1989). During the gliding process, the operator will discover contracted bands, nodules and tender points unique to that individual. Gliding repeatedly on these bands often reduces their size and tenacity, lessening the time and effort needed to modify or eliminate them. Clinical experience indicates that the best results tend to come from gliding on the tissues several times, then work-

ing somewhere else and returning to glide again. The direction of application of glides may be either with or across the direction of the muscle fibres, and usually involves a combination of both. A moist hot pack placed on the tissues between gliding repetitions further enhances the effects. A short time of rest is usual before additional gliding and allows circulatory and drainage functions to flush the tissues further. Tenderness and ischaemia are commonly rapidly reduced in this way.

The use of the hands in NMT

To most effectively glide on the tissues, the operator's hands are held with the fingers spread slightly and 'leading' the thumbs (Fig. 11.1A). The thumbs become the treatment tool while the fingers support and stabilise the hands. The hand moves as a unit with the wrist stable. Little or no motion is allowed in the wrist joint or the thumb joints. Excessive movement in the wrist or thumb may lead to joint problems and inflammation of the practitioner's forearms, wrists and hands. When two-handed glides are used, the thumbs are side by side or one ahead of the other.[2]

Speed of movement

When dealing with tissue which is not excessively tender or sensitive the 'glide' should cover 3 to 4 inches per second (speed of application is reduced for comfort if tissues are sensitive) which is significantly faster than the thumb stroke used in Lief's NMT.

It is important to develop a moderate gliding speed in order to assure adequate opportunity for simultaneous palpation of muscles. Too rapid a movement may cause unnecessary discomfort and may also skim over congestion in the tissues, missing vital information sources. Movement

---

[2]The American NMT glide is seen in this description to vary from the European hand application in which, while the fingers are placed ahead of the thumbs, they remain static while only the thumb moves during the assessment/treatment 'glide'. In the American version the whole hand moves.

that is too slow may displace the tissues, making identification of individual muscles difficult. A moderate speed will allow for repetitions which significantly increase blood flow and, at the same time, palpate bands or nodules of ischaemia within the tissues.[3]

Pressure considerations

After gliding and manipulation of tissues, the muscles may be compressed with static (ischaemic compression) pressure. Pressure should be constant and could even be mildly increased as tissues relax and release. The length of time that pressure is maintained will, however, vary but as a rule it is found that tissue contraction begins to ease within 8–12 seconds. The operator should feel the tissues 'melting and softening' under the pressure. The patient frequently reports that they believe the operator is reducing the pressure.[4]

Pain reduction not always an adequate guide

While a reduction of pain may be achieved via ischaemic compression which is sustained for longer than suggested, this is usually of only short-term benefit. Increased pain and a reduction in local mobility may result from the irritation caused by sustained or excessive pressure. A greater, longer-lasting, beneficial effect will usually be gained when the operator goes back to an area 4–5 times for 8–12 seconds than once for 40–60 seconds. If release of palpated contractions have not commenced within 8–12 seconds, the pressure may be too heavy or too light and should probably be altered.

Degree of pressure

The appropriate degree of pressure utilised in

ischaemic compression of this type varies with the individual and even from one part of the body to another. Age, oxygenation, past trauma, exercise status, previous therapies, general nutrition, mineral imbalances, tissue toxicity, and dysfunctional postures all seem to influence the amount of pressure most appropriately applied.

A 1–10 scale of discomfort in the treated tissues may be used to help guide the therapist, with 1 being no discomfort and 10 being extremely painful: a score of 5, 6 or 7 represents an ideal report, while a score of 9 or 10 has no place in therapy. 'Biting the bullet' and 'digging it out' has no advantage, and offers real disadvantages, in NMT.

Pressure bars

Pressure bars may be used as tools for treatment and are constructed of light wood. They comprise a 1 inch dowel horizontal crossbar and a $\frac{1}{4}$ inch vertical shaft and have either a $\frac{1}{2}$ inch flat rubber tip or a $\frac{1}{4}$ inch bevelled rubber tip at the end of the vertical shaft (Fig. 11.1B,C). The large flat tip is used to press into large muscle bellies, such as the gluteals or to glide on flat bellies such as the anterior tibialis. The small bevelled tip is used in the lamina groove, under the spine of the scapula and to friction certain tendons which are difficult to reach with the thumb. The bevelled end of a flat typewriter eraser can also be used. The pressure bars are never used on extremely tender tissues, at vulnerable nerve areas such as the clavicle, or to 'dig' into tissues. Contracted tissues, fibrosis, and bony surfaces may be 'felt' through the bars just as a grain of sand or a crack in the table under writing paper may be felt through a pencil when writing. The tips of the tools should be cleaned with cold sterilisation after each use. The following descriptions and illustrations of NMT applied using American methodology are not meant to be fully comprehensive; they do however provide accurate examples of the way NMT would be used were restriction being addressed and/or were trigger points being sought and treated in these structures.

---

[3]As noted in the text, NMT in Europe is usually significantly more deliberate and slow than the American version, especially in the assessment mode.
[4]The pressure applied in Lief's NMT has two distinct modes: the assessment mode 'meets and matches' tissue tension, whereas the pressure applied in NMT treatment mode is largely in accord with that described for American NMT.

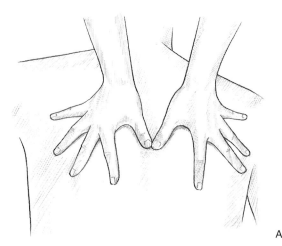

Figure 11.1A The fingers lead and steady the thumbs which are the primary tools used in most of the gliding techniques.

NMT METHODS

Trapezius

The patient lies prone with the arm hanging off the side of the table or with the hand up near the head.

1. Grasp the upper trapezius between the thumb and first three fingers with the thumb on the posterior surface and the fingers wrapping all the way around and up underneath the anterior fibres (Fig. 11.2A,B). This 'pincer' grip is suitable for this muscle as well as, with slight variations, the sternocleidomastoid and other muscles.

'Uncoil' the fibres of the outermost portion of the upper trapezius by dragging 3 fingers over the anterior surface against posteriorly applied thumb pressure. Do not allow the fingers to flip over the very edge of the trapezius as this area can be very tender with violent trigger points. Keep the wrist low to angle the fingers around the most anterior fibres. Thoroughly examine the toothpick size strands of the outermost portion which often contain trigger points which induce noxious referrals into the face and eyes.[5]

2. Place the prone patient's arm onto the table

---

[5]Lief's NMT would access these structures from a position in which the operator is at the head of the table – see position 3 of spinal NMT application in Chapter 6 (p. 96).

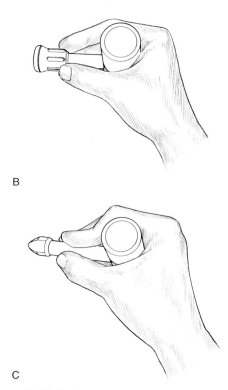

Figure 11.1B,C Pressure bars, held properly, are excellent treatment tools which relieve stress on practitioners thumbs and fingers.

at their side. Elevate the humeral head 3–6 inches (use a rolled-up towel, wedge, etc.) to shorten the middle and lower trapezius. To define the middle trapezius, draw two parallel lines from the two ends of the spine of the scapula to form right angles with the spinous processes. The middle trapezius lie between these two lines.

Grasp the middle trapezius with both hands and manipulate the belly of the middle portion (Fig. 11.2C). Repeat the grasping manipulation to the outer (diagonal) edge of the lower trapezius (Fig. 11.2D). This manipulation is similar to skin rolling techniques (see Chapter 8, p. 97, for details of skin rolling) but includes more than the skin, lifting and evaluating/stretching the fibres of the muscle itself. If trigger points are found, static pincer-like compression is used to treat them.

3. Place the small pressure bar in the lamina groove at a 45° angle against the lateral surface of the spinous processes at the level of C7.

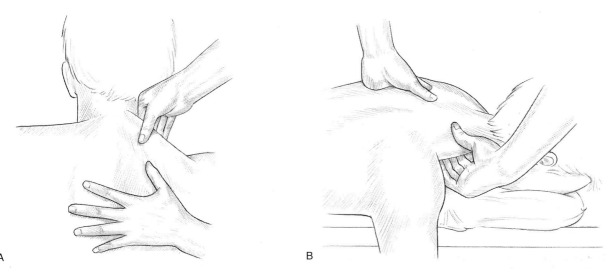

A

B

Figure 11.2A,B   Fingers should curl completely around the upper trapezius to touch the anterior surface under the forward 'lip'.

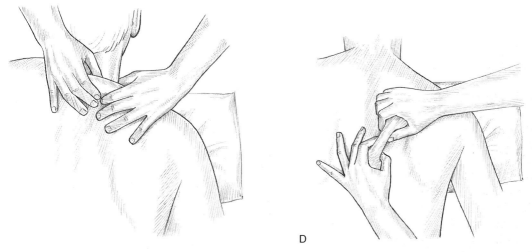

C

D

Figure 11.2C,D   Middle and lower portions of trapezius may be effectively lifted and compressed on most people by elevating the head of the humerus to shorten the fibers.

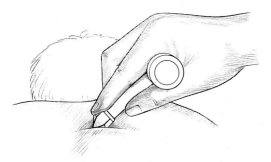

E

Figure 11.2E   The beveled pressure bar may be used in grooves and under boney ledges not easily reached with the thumbs, such as here in the spinal lamina groove.

Friction cephalad to caudad at tip width intervals all the way down to L1 to treat the trap attachments on the spinous processes as well as deeper attachments (Fig. 11.2E).[6]

4. The bevelled pressure bar may be used on the scapular and acromial attachments of the trapezius. Gliding strokes with the thumb may be used on the clavicular attachments where the pressure bar is not used.

CAUTION: It is suggested that the pressure bar not be used on clavicular attachments of the trapezius due to the proximity of the brachial plexus.

Levator scapula
(lying beneath upper trapezius)

The patient is prone.

1. Grasp the lower angle of the scapula and ease it toward the patient's ear to elevate the upper angle of the scapula away from the shoulder. The therapist's lower hand is used to increase and secure this elevation at the lower angle of the scapula (Fig. 11.3).

2. The operator's fingers of the cephalad hand are passed around the anterior fibres of the trapezius and directly onto the anterior surface of the upper angle of the scapula. It is necessary to ensure that the trapezius fibres are bypassed, since trying to access levator scapula by pressing through the trapezius fibres will fail to achieve optimal results. Friction should be lightly applied gently as these fibres are often extremely tender and can produce a dull to moderate ache in the shoulder or trapezius area. The cephalad end of these fibres attach to the atlas transverse process and are therefore involved in its stability. Gliding strokes may be applied to the remainder of the muscle and cross fibre friction at its attachments on the transverse processes of C1–C4.

Posterior mid thorax

The patient is prone.

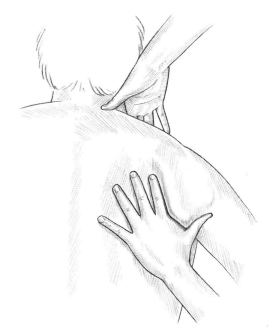

Figure 11.3 Fingers are wrapped around the anterior trapezius and placed directly on the upper angle of the manually elevated scapula to access the bony surface where levator scapula attaches.

1. Place the patient's hand behind the small of the back, if possible, so distracting the vertebral border of the scapula from the ribcage wall, allowing deeper palpation. The following steps may be more easily performed if the operator stands on the contralateral side and reaches across to apply treatment. Place the thumbs under the medial anterior surface of the scapula and introduce a glide or use cranial/caudal friction to examine the attachments of the serratus anterior and the subscapularis along the entire anterior vertebral border of the scapula (Fig. 11.4A).

2. With the scapula still elevated, place the thumbs to apply pressure anteriorly, deep to the vertebral border of the scapula, and glide or friction while pressing down onto the ribcage (Fig. 11.4B). This step will address the 'hidden' tendonous attachments of the serratus posterior superior.

Trigger points in this area significantly refer into the chest and down the arm, duplicating angina pain. They may be hidden from palpa-

---

[6]Lief's NMT would use thumb pressure to achieve the same effect.

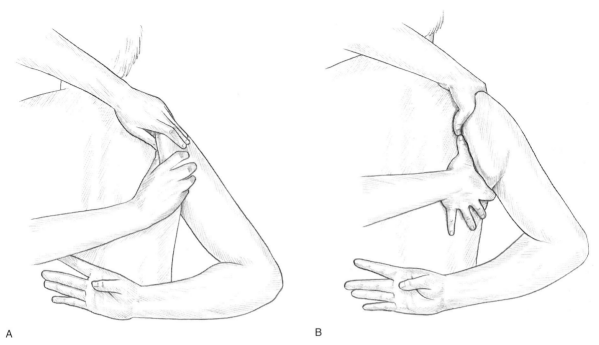

A   B

Figure 11.4A,B   'Hidden' trigger points in the posterior superior serratus may be accessed under the vertebral border of the scapula.

tion unless the scapula is sufficiently elevated.[7]

Slide in all directions between the scapulae while avoiding the spinous processes to treat several layers of muscles.

Posterior cranium

The patient is prone.

1. Carefully examine the attachments on the transverse process of C1 of the obliques capitis superior and inferior, the levator scapula and the splenius cervicis muscles (Fig. 11.5A). The SCM may need to be displaced laterally in order to palpate the muscles attaching to the transverse process of C1. The remainder of the posterior cranial attachments and the bellies of the suboccipital muscles may be treated with transverse friction from midline to the transverse process between C1 and the occiput and between C1 and C2. This suboccipital region is often involved in forward head posture and chronic headache patterns.

2. Use combination friction to examine the belly of the thin, flat occipitalis muscle which is located about 1.5 to 2 inches lateral to the occipital protuberance (Fig. 11.5B). This muscle may be palpable on some individuals when the eyebrows are raised repeatedly, since it merges with the cranial aponeurosis and connects with the frontalis muscle. Trigger points in this muscle may refer strongly into the eye and into the frontal sinus area.[8]

Cervical lamina – patient supine

1. Lubricate the lamina groove from the occiput to T1. The left hand lifts and supports the head. The right hand fingers lie across the back of the neck at the occipital ridge with the thumb placed next to the lateral surface of the spinous process of C1 (Fig. 11.6A). Glide from C1 to T1 while simultaneously pressing toward the ceiling.

---

[7]Lief's NMT would access these areas from positions 4 and 5 of the spinal sequence as described in Chapter 6 (p. 97).

[8]The position 3 of NMT spinal sequence as described in Chapter 6 (p. 96) would effectively assess and treat these structures working from the head of the table.

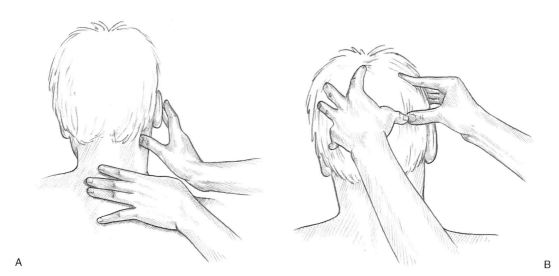

Figure 11.5A,B (A) Attachments of several muscles may be treated at the transverse process of the atlas. (B) The thin, flat occipitalis muscle refers strongly into the eye region.

Repeat the gliding movements 5–6 times. The therapist's elbow should remain low and the arm should remain in the same plane as the spine. Observe the chin moving in extension as the gliding movements of the thumb restores flexibility to the posterior cervical muscles.

2. Rotate the head away from the side being treated. Move the right thumb laterally one thumb's width (about 1 inch) and repeat the gliding movements 5–6 times (Fig. 11.6B). The chin will not move while gliding on the lateral strips.

CAUTION: Extreme head rotation is not recommended for the elderly as it may induce stress to the vertebral artery which lies within the transverse processes.

3. Continue a series of caudad glides with the thumb, moving laterally in strips until the entire lamina groove has been treated (Fig. 11.6C). Stay posterior to the transverse processes. The muscles being treated are the trapezius, semispinalis capitis, semispinalis cervicis, splenius capitis, splenius cervicis, and levator scapula.

CAUTION: It is necessary to ensure that the glides remain posterior to the transverse processes. Direct pressure onto the tips of the spinous processes is not suggested as this may traumatise tissues lying between the bony prominence and the contact thumb.

4. Return to any ischaemic bands or trigger points found and treat with static compression.[9]

Splenii tendons

1. **CAUTION**: Use no pressure until the thumb is securely in place as described below.

To treat the right side splenius capitis, the patient is supine and the operator's right hand fingers cup across the back of the neck like a shirt collar. Place the right thumb anterior to the trapezius and posterior to the transverse processes, while pointing the thumb toward the patient's feet. Use the left hand to rotate the head toward the side being treated (Fig. 11.7A).

2. The right hand should rotate with the neck as if moulded to the back of the neck. This rotation will open a 'pocket' anterior to the trapezius, allowing the thumb to be angled toward the nipple of the opposite breast, pressing

---

[9]Lief's NMT would have accessed these areas alongside the cervical spine with the patient prone, in positions 1, 2, 3, 4 and 5 of the spinal sequence as described in Chapter 6 (pp. 94–97). Direct strokes over the tips of the spinous processes are included in this sequence but caution is suggested so that pressure remain light. The interspinous spaces commonly house trigger points and the attachments to the spinous processes themselves may manifest as periosteal pain points, indicating a need for attention from the muscles which are producing the stress.

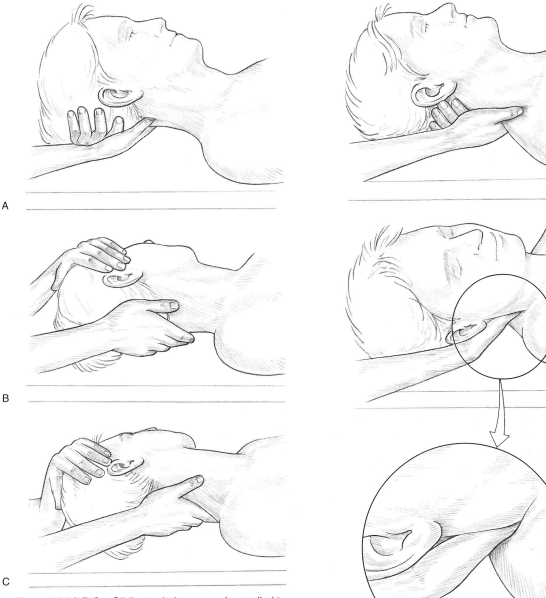

Figure 11.6A,B,C   Gliding techniques may be applied to the cervical lamina from the occiput to the thorax as far laterally as the transverse processes.

Figure 11.7A,B,C   Originally called the corkscrew technique by Dr. Nimmo, treatment of the splenii tendons from C7-T4 is applied 'in the pocket' anterior to the trapezius.

lightly against the lateral surface of the spinous processes (Fig. 11.7B,C). The thumb pad should now be facing toward the ceiling. Slide the right thumb into the 'pocket' formed by the trapezius. If the 'pocket' does not allow penetration of the thumb due to excessive tension, or if pressure of the thumb produces more than moderate dis-

comfort, press lightly at the 'mouth' of the pocket until the tissues relax enough to slide in further.

3. Apply pressure towards the lateral surface

of the spinous processes and simultaneously toward the ceiling for 8–12 seconds. The thumb will be pressing into the tendons of the splenius capitis and splenius cervicis as well as the deeper muscles of the rotatores and multifidi. After the initial application of pressure, rest for a few seconds and then press the thumb into the pocket a little deeper and repeat the manoeuvre. When the tissues prevent the thumb's caudad movements, mild to moderate static pressure may produce more opening of the pocket and allow the therapist to go a little further down the spinal column.

4. If tender, repeat the entire process 3–4 times during a session. This step will help restore cervical rotation as well as reduce tilting pull on the transverse processes of C1–3. Trigger points in the splenii tendons can refer strongly into the eye, causing eye pressure-like discomfort. Operators should rule out glaucoma or other serious eye conditions as a cause of such discomfort, in addition to treating these tissues.

Sternocleidomastoid

The release of the sternocleidomastoid muscle is important because of its propensity to distract the head anteriorly. Compensating postural distortions relating to such forward head positions can include anterior rotation of the pelvis, reversed or straightened thoracic curve as well as changes in cervical lordosis. Trigger points in this muscle can cause severe eye pain, temporomandibular joint pain, sore throat, hearing loss or ear pain, and can mimic migraine headaches.

The patient is supine.

1. Do not lubricate the tissues but grasp the tendon of the SCM lightly between the thumb and first two fingers as close to the mastoid process as possible. Rotate the head toward the side being treated to rotate it away from the carotid artery. Tilt (side-bend) the head toward the side being treated to more easily grasp the SCM and so lift it away from the deeper tissues (Fig. 11.8A). Be sure to grasp both heads of the SCM. A paper tissue may help the grasp if the area is oily.

CAUTION: If a pulse from the carotid artery is noted while compressing the SCM release the muscle immediately and reposition the fingers to ensure the artery is not compressed.

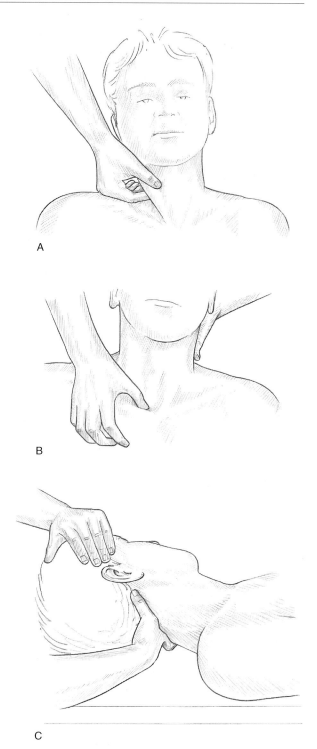

A

B

C

Figure 11.8A,B,C   Thorough treatment of the sternocleidomastoid often relieves symptoms associated with migraine headaches, temporomandibular joint dysfunction and hearing problems. (C) Longissimus capitus and splenius capitus may be reached under the posterior aspect of the mastoid attachement of SCM.

2. Compress the SCM for 8–12 seconds at 1 inch intervals from the mastoid process to the sternal and clavicular attachments. Each head can be treated separately. Medial to lateral friction may be used on the sternal and clavicular attachments (Fig. 11.8B).

3. Support the head at a 45° of flexion and rotate it away from the side being treated. Glide inferiorly on the upper 1 inch of the mastoid attachment of the SCM while being careful to avoid the styloid process located anterior to it.

4. Place the thumb posterior to the SCM tendon at the mastoid process and displace the tendon anteriorly while simultaneously pressing onto the mastoid attachment of the longissimus capitis (erector spinae) and the splenius capitis. Use static pressure or combination friction to treat them (Fig. 11.8C).[10]

Spinal lamina groove

Trigger points lying close to the lamina of the spinal column often refer pain across the back, wrapping around the rib cage, anteriorly into the chest or abdomen and frequently refer 'itching' patterns. The treatment technique described below is particularly useful if scoliosis is evident.

Technique: 1. Angle a small pressure bar at 45° against the lateral surface of the spinous processes (Fig. 11.9A,B). Use caudad/cephalad friction at tip-width intervals from C7 to the coccyx on each side of each segment. Avoid pressure with the bar on the coccyx.

2. When moving the pressure bar lift it and place it at the next site to avoid gliding it as the small bevelled head may cause tissue irritation. Avoid treating the cervical lamina with the pressure bar as the cervical vertebrae are less stable than those below C7.

3. Friction may also be performed between spinous processes with the small bar in order to treat interspinalis muscles and the supraspinous ligament (Fig. 11.9C).[11]

---

[10]Lief's NMT would access and treat dysfunction in these structures with the patient prone, from positions 1, 2, 3 of the sequence described in Chapter 6 (pp. 92–98).
[11]Lief's spinal NMT application addresses these tissues with thumb and/or finger contacts as described in Chapter 6 (p. 96).

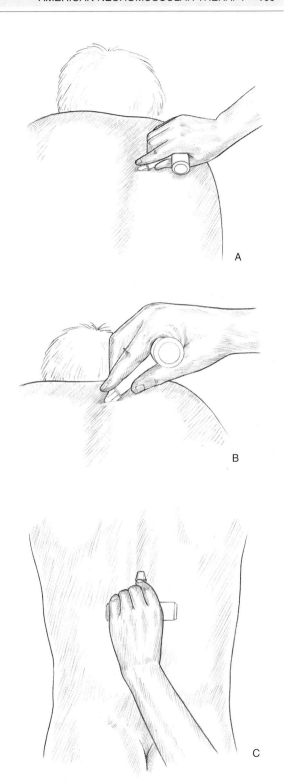

A

B

C

Figure 11.9A,B,C The small beveled pressure bar may be used the entire length of the spine and sacrum, both in the lamina (A, B) and between the spinous processes (C). The cervical region should not be treated with the tool.

Intercostal muscles

1. Place the small pressure bar inferior to the clavicle of the supine patient, just lateral to the sternum, in the first intercostal space (Fig. 11.10A).

The bevelled tip should lie between the ribs and parallel with them. Using medial/lateral friction at each application site move the bar laterally at tip intervals until pectoralis minor is reached.

2. Return to the sternum and move down one rib space and repeat the tip width examination while using frictional pressure as described in 1. above until pectoralis minor is reached. Avoid pressure into pectoralis minor as there are sensitive neural structures in the area.

3. Avoid contact with breast tissue. When working around the breast, use the person's hand to displace the breast away from the treatment site inferiorly, laterally, superiorly or medially as appropriate in order to allow access for the pressure bar to the intercostal under examination/treatment.

4. Continue the intercostal work as far caudad and laterally as possible using a side-lying position, which allows access to the more lateral aspects of the intercostal spaces (Fig. 11.10B,C).

5. With the patient prone, place the pressure bar into the intercostal space lateral to the first thoracic vertebra. With the bevel parallel to the ribs and the rib space, use medial/lateral friction at width-tip intervals in the same manner as that applied on the anterior surface.

Continue the treatment in all intercostal spaces as far caudad and laterally as possible.[12] Distinction of the rib spaces may be difficult in the upper thorax where superficial tissue is thicker.

---

[12]Lief's NMT would access the intercostal spaces from the mid-axillary line to the spine, using finger-tip pressure while treating the prone patient, as described in Chapter 6 (positions 4, 5, 6 and 7, pp. 98–101). Anterior intercostal evaluation and treatment would be performed as appropriate with the patient supine as illustrated in Chapter 7 (lower intercostal only described and illustrated, pp. 105–106) relating to abdominal application of NMT. The same cautions discussed in the text in this chapter would be issued for manual as for pressure bar applications in the intercostal tissues.

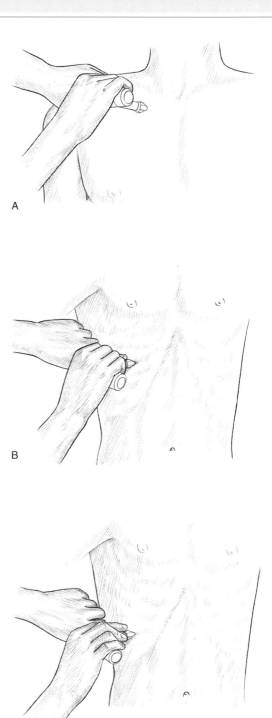

A

B

C

Figure 11.10A,B,C The small beveled bar may be used at tip width intervals throughout each intercostal space, especially on people with respiratory ailments. Avoid pressing on the brachial plexus or breast tissue.

Iliolumbar ligament and sacroiliac ligament

1. In order to treat the iliolumbar ligament using NMT, a thumb is placed on the posterior superior iliac spine (PSIS) and the index finger of the same hand is placed on the spinous process of L5 (Fig. 11.11A). The other hand holds the large pressure bar and this is pressed directly towards the floor into the tissue between the two contact digits (Fig. 11.11B). The bar should press into the superficial tissue above the ligament and should not make any osseous contact on the sacrum. If it does it should be moved slightly cephalad until it is in contact with soft tissue only. The pressure is held for 8 to 12 seconds in order to apply ischaemic compression to the overlying muscles and the ligament itself.

2. The same contact should then be re-examined with the small pressure bar, with the bevel held parallel to the crest of the ilium. It should be moved medially to the quadratus lumborum until contact is made with the iliolumbar ligament. A cross fibre movement is used with the bevelled tip while it is angled to access the tissues anterior to the lateral edge of the erector spinae muscles (Fig. 11.11C).

3. In order to treat the sacroiliac ligament using NMT, the small pressure bar is held and placed at a 45° angle onto the lateral aspect of the sacral tubercles (Fig. 11.12A). Commencing at the cephalad aspect of the sacrum a cephalad/caudad frictional movement is introduced in order to examine the tissues. The pressure bar is then moved one tip width caudad and the friction is repeated. This continues up to the coccyx, which should not itself receive any treatment of this sort.

4. Returning to the sacral base, the pressure bar is applied into the soft tissues one tip-width laterally to the initial contact, at 90° to the surface (i.e. to the dorsum of the sacrum) (Fig. 11.12B). The procedure as above is then repeated until the coccyx is reached. In this way the entire sacral dorsal surface should be treated in 'strips'. No pressure should be applied onto the ilium or to the tissues lateral to the border of the sacrum.

A uniform pattern should be visible with no

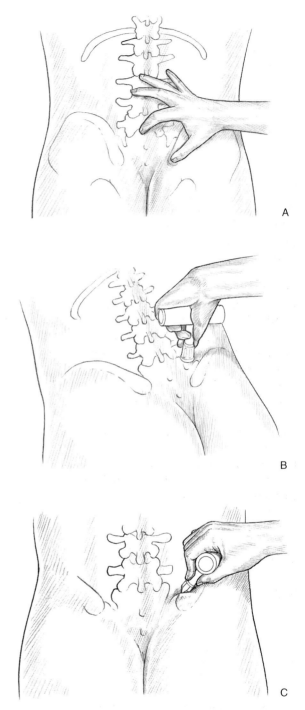

Figure 11.11A,B,C The iliolumbar ligament, located between the spinous process of L5 and the posterior superior iliac spine and just above the sacrum, can be treated through the erector spinae (B) or under its lateral edge (C).

while gradually increasing pressure in order to relax and warm the tissues (Fig. 11.13A).

2. Standing at waist level with the forward foot at shoulder level and the back foot at waist level, facing towards the head with knees slight-

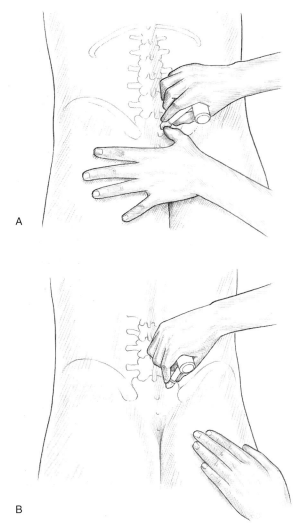

Figure 11.12A,B If not inflammed, the entire surface of the sacrum can be treated to address sacroiliac ligaments as well as multifidus and erector spinae attachments. Trigger points here will refer sciatica-like pain.

gaps between the prints left by the tip pressure applications. All the strips of prints should be parallel to the sacral tubercles.

Erector spinae

1. The erector spinae muscles should be lubricated from C7 to the sacrum. The thumbs or palm are used to glide along this pathway (C7 to sacrum) repeatedly, alternating from side to side

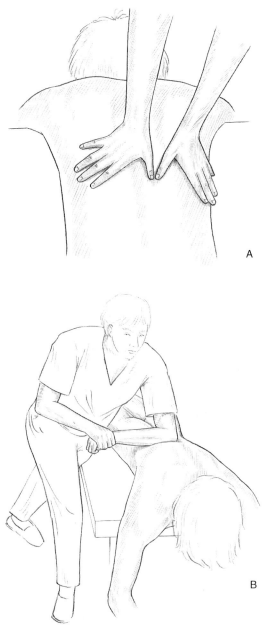

Figure 11.13A,B Long, gliding strips, applied with the thumbs, palms, fists or forearm, lengthen thoracic fascia while treating several layers of muscles.

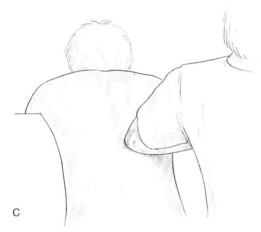

C

Figure 11.13C   When working near the spine, avoid pressing on spinous processes.

ly flexed, the olecranon process of the tableside elbow is placed against but not onto the spinous processes at the level of L5 (Fig. 11.13B). With a moderate pressure and speed, the entire length of the paraspinal tissues, including the erector spinae, receive the benefit of a glide from this contact. The pressure should be moderated when the thoracic region is being traversed. Modification of the angle of contact will be necessary when covering the erector spinae medial to the scapulae. Care should be taken not to apply pressure onto the spinous processes themselves (Fig. 11.13C). End the stroke at C7 and use thumbs in the cervical region.

3. Turn to face the feet and apply forearm contact to the erector spinae as a series of glides are performed from C7 to the iliac crest. No pressure should be applied in this way onto the iliac crest itself or the sacrum.

4. The thumbs, or knuckles, or the large pressure bar may be used to cautiously cross-fibre the long tendons of the erectors; however, the spinous processes should not be involved in these contacts.[13]

Quadratus lumborum

1. After application of a lubricant, a glide up quadratus lumborum is made using both thumbs, from the crest of the ilium to the 12th rib. The initial contact remains just lateral to the erector spinae as 4 or 5 repetitious glides are applied to the medial aspect of the muscle (Fig. 11.14A). The thumbs are then placed approximately an inch laterally and the glides are repeated. A series of glides are then performed, in 'strips', moving laterally until the entire muscle has been treated. If necessary, by moving more lateral still, the obliques can be treated as well.

2. Facing the feet of the prone patient, standing at chest level, glide caudad from the 12th rib to the crest of the ilium, ensuring that contact is lateral to the erector spinae. A series of glides moving laterally is then performed (Fig. 11.14B).

3. Facing the head, and with the fingers of the lateral hand moulded around the curve of the trunk and the thumb angled at 45° to the spine, the thumb is glided medially on the inferior surface of the 12th rib until it reaches the lateral aspect of the erector spinae. In order to avoid trauma, no pressure should be applied onto the lateral aspect of the transverse processes in this region, which are located just lateral to the lateral border of the erector spinae. Apply static pressure or friction on posterior aspect of the transverse process of L1. Follow this with similar applications of friction or pressure onto the lumbar transverse processes at 1 to 2 inch intervals down to the level of L4 (Fig. 11.14C).[14]

Overview of differences

The key variations existing between the European (Lief's) and the American versions of NMT – which emerge from these examples – seem to relate to a far more structured and prescriptive approach in American NMT, with a variety of

---

[13]Lief's NMT attention to these same tissues forms a major element of the approach described in Chapter 6, most notably in relation to positions 3, 4, 5, 6, 7, 8 and 9 (pp. 92–101), where thumb and/or finger strokes would be the main means of contact.

[14]Lief's NMT would access these tissues from positions 8 and 9 of the spinal application as described in Chapter 6 (p. 100).

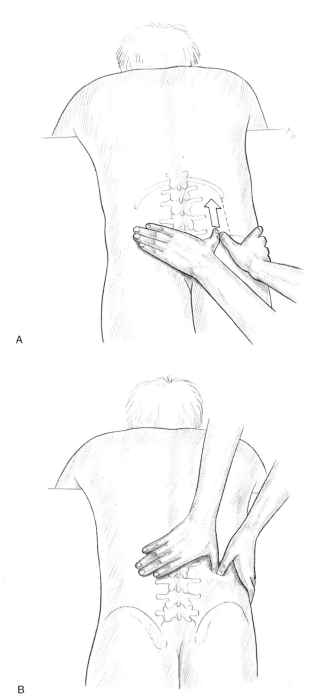

A

B

Figure 11.14A,B The quadratus lumborum will be treated lateral to the erector spinae by gliding between the crest of the ilium and the last rib.

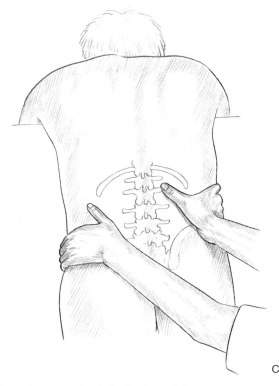

C

Figure 11.14C Quadratus lumborum's transverse process attachments may be felt on some people just lateral to the erector spinae. L2 and L3 are palpable on most people. L1 and L4 may be more difficult to locate.

additional 'tools' being used – including elbows and pressure bars. While Lief's version also has a (different) structured outline it seems to require fewer 'strokes' or 'glides', remaining in assessment mode until something is discovered which calls for therapeutic input. At that time, apart from the more restricted variety of contacts, relying almost solely on finger or thumb contact, the way in which tissues are addressed, using ischaemic compression and frictional or cross fibre methods, seems very similar to the American method.

American NMT seems to move directly into a therapeutic 'glide' which has assessment potential, while Lief's approach separates assessment from therapeutic input more definitively.

REFERENCES

Cailliet R 1977 Soft tissue pain and disability. F A Davis, Philadelphia

Travell J, Simons D 1983 Myofascial pain and dysfunction, (vol 1) Williams and Wilkins, Baltimore

Vannerson J, Nimmo R 1971 Specificity and the law of facilitation in the nervous system. The Receptor 2(1)

Yates J 1989 Physiological effects of therapeutic massage and their application to treatment. Massage Therapy Association of British Columbia, Vancouver

Index